DISABILITY IS OTHER PEOPLE
MY SUPERHERO STORY

DISABILITY IS OTHER PEOPLE

MY SUPERHERO STORY

Richard C Brown MBE

Copyright © 2024 Richard C Brown MBE

The moral right of the author has been asserted.

Apart from any fair dealing for the purposes of research or private study, or criticism or review, as permitted under the Copyright, Designs and Patents Act 1988, this publication may only be reproduced, stored or transmitted, in any form or by any means, with the prior permission in writing of the publishers, or in the case of reprographic reproduction in accordance with the terms of licences issued by the Copyright Licensing Agency. Enquiries concerning reproduction outside those terms should be sent to the publishers.

Troubador Publishing Ltd
Unit E2 Airfield Business Park
Harrison Road, Market Harborough
Leicestershire LE16 7UL
Tel: 0116 279 2299
Email: books@troubador.co.uk
Web: www.troubador.co.uk

ISBN 978-1-80514-449-6

British Library Cataloguing in Publication Data.
A catalogue record for this book is available from the British Library.

Printed and bound in Great Britain by 4edge Limited
Typeset in 11pt Acumin Pro by Troubador Publishing Ltd, Leicester, UK

For Helen, Bella, Billy, Treacle & Tara –
Best Family Ever!

CONTENTS

Introduction IX

Part One: Real Gone Kid 1
Part Two: Rise 67
Part Three: A Day In The Life 115
Part Four: (Just Like) Starting Over 181
Part Five: Times Like These 249
Part Six: Gimme Some Truth 303

The Takeaway 344

Acknowledgements 349
Bibliography 350

INTRODUCTION

Superheroes are everywhere these days; they're in our stories, memories and legends, our dreams and nightmares. They are in our very bones.

Our modern idea of 'the superhero' (Morris, 2005) began with a philosopher named Nietzsche. He believed that the *Ubermench,* or Superman, was someone who masters their own fate by rejecting societal and cultural norms and follows their own will.

This idea developed through the comics of the late '30s which began to show stories of heroes with extraordinary powers, like DC's Superman. At the same time, the idea was popular with Nazi ideology, but died with the Third Reich. His ideas of God and man remain an important part of how we see ourselves. Today's *Marvel* franchise has introduced us to a complex range of mutants, gods, and monsters. The series of X-MEN films developed the idea of people with extraordinary powers and abilities. Such people are quickly surrounded by fear, suspicion and discrimination. Made to feel sub-human, they are labelled as 'mutants' and forced out of society. Filmlifestyle.com describes a superhero as one 'who has exceptional abilities or powers, either acquired naturally or through science. They use those abilities to fight crime and do good in the world.' But wait, this also describes disabled people!

We're all battling our own supernatural impairments. You may not have realised, but disabled people are fighting on your behalf every day. We fight through a universe of constant battles against a mostly ignorant or hostile society, institutions that are supposed to support us, and service providers who are supposed to provide inclusive services. We protect the public by calling for our society to be a fairer, more accessible place – the kind you will need when disability comes to you. We know what being different feels like.

Now, what else do disabled people and superheroes have in common? Both have an origin story.

An origin story is a storytelling tradition that gives readers clues about how a character sees and interacts with the world around them. The *Superhero Reader* (Hatfield, 2013) explains that the value of 'stories about destroyed worlds, murdered parents, genetic mutations, and mysterious power-giving wizards is to realize the degree to which the superhero genre is about transformation, about identity, about difference, and about the tension between psychological rigidity and a flexible and fluid sense of human nature.'

You could say that a simple genetic mutation changed my life, but 'Holy wheelchairs, Batman!'. Transformation, identity and difference – this is what disability is about too! Our society definitely understands both disabled people and superheroes in the same ways! Does that mean I'm a superhero?

Let me tell you my origin story ...

I was just an ordinary 14-year-old, discovering music and girls, when I first noticed a deep, painful, and chronic tiredness – the kind you can't shake off with a good rest and some paracetamol. I underwent tests; shocking, painful tests. A consultant gave me an equally painful diagnosis: Friedreich's ataxia, a progressive and incurable genetic condition that would cause the gradual loss of motor function, leading to wheelchair use, and early death. I was devastated. I longed for my own family, my own home, and my own career, which I could now never have. I hoped to go to university, to drive, and to travel, which I could never do. Heartbroken, I dropped out of school and spent the next few years drifting aimlessly. Totally lost. Then I met Helen and she believed in me. Somehow, she saw my potential when I had given up on myself. Now, some 30 years later, thanks mainly to hard work and grim determination, I can proudly say that I overcame this terrible affliction as well as doing all those things I dreamed of, and so much more.

Yes, that is *kind of* my origin story, but telling it feels too simple. I repeat it often because it is what other people expect to hear. It fits the common narrative that most people understand and accept when thinking about disabled people – the tragedy. This story has all the right ingredients: an innocent encountering terrible misfortune, a struggle, and overcoming eye-watering odds to triumph.

This story, then, is what I think other people expect. I understand their curiosity in 'what happened to me', but it also strengthens the 'othering' of disabled people. It supports the ableist ideas that we are broken, doomed to struggle and that our lives have no value. I believe that this narrative is created, accepted and perpetuated by society as a simple way to understand disability. I first used the phrase 'disability is other people' in 2016 to describe it. Taken from the Jean-Paul Sartre's existential play: *No Exit* (Satre, 2013). A character, trapped with two others in a room in hell with no windows or doors, soon realises that hell is actually being trapped with other people. I think this shows that negative ideas of disability are created and perpetuated by other people.

On hearing my experience, people are moved; they tell me I am brave or an inspiration. I know I have hit the mark. I believe that by exploiting my story to manipulate the listener, to extract sympathy and admiration, I do myself and other disabled people a great disservice. Acting more like a supervillain, I have reinforced all the common stereotypes that

Introduction

disabled people struggle against! I become part of the problem. Disability is much more complex and can be surprisingly positive. We can change these attitudes by telling our own stories.

Stories and storytelling fascinate me, but that one is shallow and effortless. It does not capture the whole truth – my truth. This is my story. It has some similarities, then again also more complexities. It is a story about other people. The ones who made a difference. I bat-promise you that this journey will be much more interesting.

Above all, this version of the story is anything but a tragedy. Maybe there are tragic moments for our hero (me) to deal with… but really this story is an odyssey, a search for meaning amid the victories and defeats of trying to be a superhero. My quest begins with Part One, where I share my origins, my early years and teens, and how I faced my diagnosis and the emptiness that followed. In Part Two, I introduce you to my amazing wife, Helen, and how my life changed at university. In Part Three, I tell you how I pursued my career and became a parent, slowly achieving all the things I never thought possible. In Part Four, I recount how an unexpected early retirement led me to volunteer and discover the true meaning and purpose of life. In Part Five, I reflect on how the Covid-19 pandemic changed everything, gave me the opportunity to re-evaluate myself and my place in the world. In Part Six, I bring everything together and suggest just why our society lets disabled people down so badly, and what we have to do to change it.

Why share my story now? I'm finding it more of a challenge to manage a big project like this. The whole writing process has been like a never-ending blog post, with so many thoughts, ideas, and messages that need to be expressed and linked together. I want to get it done while I can still enjoy it, and before it becomes too much of a struggle. Writing honestly about yourself and focusing on the important information can be challenging. Due to my love of reading, writing, and history, I have always written about my experiences, sometimes recycling them through essays, talks or through my blog. I have used this rich seam of writing to throw some light on some of my memories. You're getting the truth, at least as I remember it. As I put the cartoon panels of my story together, I realised that the way I saw and experienced events in life wasn't necessarily the same as other people who were there too, so I apologise to anyone I have forgotten or misrepresented.

When I stepped down as a Trustee of Ataxia UK after eight years, I saw there were plenty of younger people eager to replace me who reminded me of myself when I started. My older and wiser self could see how my role in the ataxia community was changing, so I thought 'Maybe now is a good time to look back. Older people write their memoirs and pass on their wisdom, don't they?' Most importantly, I want to leave something for my beloved family, as

I accept that I may not be with them for as long as we'd all like.

I hope this book will be of use to people like me, coming to terms with a new and frightening condition, and for their wider family and allies. The stories I share show everything I learned through my triumphs and mistakes. I would be happy if this work helps anyone feeling alone and scared. I've been in that dark place myself. So here's a friendly voice with some advice on how disability works and how to come to peace with it.

This is not the story of me becoming a superhero; instead, it's the much more personal and interesting story of how I learned what disability really is and where it comes from and that being a superman in the eyes of society is impossible.

Enjoy ...

Part One

Real Gone Kid

My story doesn't really begin with aching muscles at 14. It starts well before then. I once knew what it was to live a 'normal' life.

ORIGINS

In my early years, I thought I had special powers. I knew exactly what grown-ups wanted and was very good at avoiding trouble. Sometimes, adults would see through this secret power. In Grandma's busy kitchen one Sunday afternoon – cool terracotta floor tiles, with steel saucepan lids rattling on the hob, the air full of steam and the smell of roasting meat – she turned and asked if I had been playing around the coal bunker. 'No,' I answered, looking her straight in the eye, using all my charm. Of course I had been playing near the coal bunker. I was at that stage of fearless exploring and squeezing my body into the tightest places I could find. I didn't know it at the time, but I was covered in cobwebs, my face streaked with coal dust. To my barefaced lie, Grandma replied coolly, 'I suppose butter wouldn't melt in your mouth?' I had never heard this expression before and tried to guess the right answer, the right thing to say. Logic told me butter would melt in my mouth, or was I being accused of taking some? 'No,' I replied again, looking down sadly, thinking I had got away with it.

Both my parents came from backgrounds that, for different reasons, offered little prospect of advancement. My dad was the son of Irish immigrants who came to Birmingham from Dublin after the war. His father, also called Robert, worked at Snow Hill station until it closed as a freight depot, and then worked night shifts in a factory in Aston, Birmingham. He drank heavily and gambled too much. For my dad, giving us what he never had was important, with an emphasis on comfort over ambition. As part of a lively Irish community, he lived with his parents and his three brothers in a terraced house in Aston. Like many working-class youths of his generation he was a teenager before the house had hot water and an inside toilet.

My mum's background was a little more affluent. Her older sister went to university! As with many families in post-war Britain, having a career outside motherhood was an exception. Originally from Staffordshire and Derbyshire, her family worked in local industries throughout the nineteenth century, such as pottery, farming, mining, brewing, and glassmaking. My mum's parents had lived on the edge of their means. Not using credit, rather living in a nice house in a nice area and secretly just getting by. My grandma, Irene, was given a strict weekly allowance to run the house and clothe the children. Appearances were very important.

My mum's father, Wilfred, did not wait to be conscripted when the Second World War came. He volunteered to join the RAF and served in North Africa as ground crew. His training manuals still survive: page after page of technical drawings of aeroplane parts and engine components, with his own careful notes covering them. He took his job very seriously and worked very hard at it.

For him, the war changed the world he came back to. He would not have 'messed about with foreign food' at his table and was hard on his family, keeping a strictly disciplined home. During the war, his wife had returned to her job as a manageress in a department store. She must've resented his return and her return to domestic slavery. An ambulance superintendent up to his fatal heart attack, he died shortly before I was born. Grandma wrote poetry throughout her life, and spoke of Wilfred as a principled and steadfast husband in her later years.

My dad was a great admirer of American folk music, especially Bob Dylan, and, as he was a few years older than my mum, was able to use this and his inner-city credentials to come across as mysterious, more experienced, and worldlier. After all, he had seen Dylan at the Isle of Wight Festival in 1969. My mum was selling Golden Goal Tickets when she met my dad on the terraces of Villa Park. Each ticket represented one second of the match; you were a winner if the time on your ticket matched the timing of the first goal. Two things have always impressed me about this meeting. Firstly, that my parents chose each other out of a crowd of thousands. Secondly, that he never even bought a ticket! You've gotta buy a ticket! (You'll see why later.) When they started seeing each other and my dad met his future father-in-law, the world had hurtled forward enough so that the young apprentice lift engineer from Birmingham was already earning more than his future father-in-law.

CHILDHOOD

I was born on the 13th of March 1976 at about ten-thirty on a Saturday evening, in Marston Green Maternity Hospital, Birmingham. Born on the 13th, living at number 13 and receiving 13 welcome cards ... that was a sign of something, surely? The idea that I was a special child had started.

For my dad, however, *Match of the Day* had just started when he was called to see his new son. I imagine him looking mournfully at the muted hospital television as he followed the nurse to the ward. Despite goals from Ray Graydon and Andy Grey, Tottenham had climbed above Villa with a 5-2 win, leaving them perilously near the bottom of the division with only a handful of games to go. If they needed a superhero, I had arrived just in time!

I was brought back to our house in Alum Rock, inner-city Birmingham, and initiated into the Brown/

Russell family with plenty of attention and indulgence. This was one of the hottest summers on record. Rivers had dried up, and swarms of ladybirds roamed the country seeking food. My arrival was a welcome distraction from the heat, as well as Grandma's recent bereavement. Reminiscent of another time, she was a model of hospitality and creativity; she wrote poetry, decorated cakes (both to a professional standard), and made everything from scratch. How I loved the teas and Sunday roasts at her house! She held them in the front room (reserved for special occasions), where we savoured succulent roast lamb or beef with home-grown seasonal veg and finished with a crumble. For tea: a myriad of sandwiches, cakes, and other desserts. Butterfly cakes filled with smooth and sweet buttercream, trifle and cheesecake. These evenings were magical affairs. Everything was home-made and to a professional standard, but these events were also a clear aspirational statement.

As an after-dinner treat, hungry for tales of wartime adventure and daring, I was allowed to browse my grandfather's wartime photos, kept in an old ammo tin. I was also curious to know about the man whose oddly cold presence was still all around us in the house. One picture I remember was of 20 young men in German uniform packed into the dark fuselage of a plane, grinning at the photographer like superheroes. Even then, I could feel this was a significant moment in time for those young men and I wondered what their story was.

I learned years later that Wilfred was attached to an aircraft recovery and salvage unit in North Africa. He would arrive on the scene of a plane crash and would comb it for parts for salvage, or hunt for intelligence and destroy the wreckage. He also collected the personal effects. His role would have often taken his unit well behind enemy lines and they would have been expected to defend themselves while about it. He had a very dangerous job. Like many, he never talked about it. Salvaging would have utilised his high-level understanding of aircraft engines. This must be how he found the picture, undeveloped inside its camera. It was probably the last photo that was ever taken of these men before their plane crashed.

The atmosphere of respectability that surrounded Grandma's house was very much enhanced by her son's presence. Everyone has a 'funny' uncle. I'm proud to say that mine is Uncle Brian. Like an Edwardian gentleman, his appearance and manners were impeccable. Like Grandma, he appeared to be someone from a different time. An eccentric and amusing man, as uncles are meant to be. Having worked in the hospitality industry, he would serve exotic-sounding liqueurs (Tia Maria, Dubonnet, Kahlúa, etc.) in special crystal glasses from a tray after dinner. He lived at Walsall Road with Grandma – eventually becoming her carer and moving with her to a flat in Lichfield when the house became too much for her. A big-hearted soul, he has always been kind and generous to all his nieces and nephews.

Occasionally we would go to Nanny's house in Aston, Birmingham. This darkened, terraced house with its mysterious rooms and narrow passageways was a world away from Grandma's respectable house in Lichfield; it was very much a living house. My grandad, Bob, would watch the wrestling, racing or the football results with me on his lap. Two of my dad's younger brothers, Ken and Chris, came and went. As Irish hospitality insists, there was always as much strong, dark tea as you could drink. I don't remember any cooked meals. In stark contrast to mealtimes in Lichfield, Dad would go down to the chip shop to get dinner, while Mum and Nanny prepared the bread and butter. I didn't pay much attention to the conversation, but I'm sure that much of it revolved around what a dangerous and unpleasant place Birmingham was becoming. This was directly attributable to Enoch Powell's hate-filled 'rivers of blood' speech in Birmingham just 15 years earlier. To emphasise this, heavy curtains blocked out the daylight from every window and a musty smell hung inside the house.

My uncles would return from this dangerous world outside and have hushed conversations with my dad. Ken especially would only give mysterious and evasive answers to my extensive questions as to his whereabouts. They were denizens of an underworld, and the mystery excited me. Several years before, Grandad told my dad an old family story that added to this air of mystery. He said that the Brown family name was made up by an individual who wanted to evade recriminations for his part in a maritime tragedy. True enough, that branch of the family tree first appears in 1917, with the mysterious Henry Brown being recorded as living in Scotland on his son's wedding certificate.

As our family grew, we escaped Birmingham and moved to a modern three-bedroom house in Mum's home town of Lichfield. It was just 20 miles away, but it was far enough. My parents had mortgaged themselves as heavily as possible, deciding that getting out of Birmingham was a positive, upward move, and worth significant debt. Dad was working in Birmingham, so he would commute by train, cycling to the station and keeping contact with head office by various telephone boxes.

Bob died from a fall at home when I was five. I think Nanny withdrew into herself after that. It was like it was too late for them to get out of Birmingham as the strength and desire for that fight had gone. There were Irish neighbours and family and friends nearby; their numbers were slowly decreasing as they moved to the edges of Birmingham or retired and returned to Ireland. The Browns seemed to be stuck, like they were watching the tide going out, slowly receding. The barriers went up. I remember waiting outside the house in the family car for Nanny, who didn't have a phone, to come and let us in. Still, Nanny repeatedly warned my dad that his children had to be looked after and kept out of Birmingham at all costs.

The first challenge to my specialness was my younger brother. I didn't deal with a new addition to the family very well. Not only was he younger than me – 16 months is a lot when you are small – we were, and still are, totally different people. As a child, he was quick to cry and prone to violent tantrums. He didn't fit into the way I wanted to be seen by people – appearances being important. He held me back. I needed attention and he represented a loss of parental attention. I was intensely jealous. I soon realised that Anthony did not have the same affinity with adults as me. He could never emulate my charm, and I could even play off him. I remember playing with the neighbour's children, for example, where usually the game was to run away from Anthony. I assumed this was how all older brothers felt about their siblings. We found it impossible to be friends; we were divided by our different needs for attention, our different personalities, and the age gap. We were able to co-operate, but very rarely. Consequently, both of us sought any advantage that we could over the other. Mum remembers that Anthony and I responded quite differently to being ill as young children. I would want constant reassurance and he would not.

One morning, my brother and I were ushered to the front window, still yawning and in pyjamas. Outside sat a dark blue Hillman Hunter with four doors. Dad had been to collect it the night before. Until then we used Dad's work van as a family vehicle, with seats from a Mini tied down between the wheel arches. This was a fantastic way to travel. The back seats were accessed by clambering over those at the front, and there were no windows. The interior of the van was occasionally illuminated by the tail lights, as Dad braked or indicated. His oily tools covered by old curtains.

To complete the eclectic social spectrum of these childhood visits were less frequent trips to my mum's sister and her husband. Angela and Peter had children of similar ages to the three of us and lived in a big house in a leafy commuter suburb outside London. Angela would take us on exciting sightseeing trips and to galleries and museums in London. My mum and her big sister were close. For me, the only difference between them was that Angela and Peter had done well for themselves. They went abroad for holidays, and their children would attend the best schools, learn Latin and archery and were destined to run the country one day. My cousins were on a very different trajectory to mine. I would feel pressure to prove that a bright, intelligent child could equally be the product of a state education as a private school.

This cosy world was shaken by my first experience of death. I was only 4 when John Lennon was assassinated. I was familiar with all the songs from his album, *Imagine*. I was also aware that his songs were amazingly powerful and expressive, and at the same time they showed Lennon at his most vulnerable. He held the status of a poet and a guru for my parents and was someone that they had grown up with as a cultural reference point. I remember seeing that they were deeply shocked, and asked them: 'What has happened to your hero?', 'Where has he gone?', and 'Is he coming back?' More than a death, this had been a violent murder. Bad things were not supposed to happen to people that my parents loved. The image of his shattered and twisted spectacles in a pool of blood in the press overstated what was already a terrible loss. A hefty cosmic lesson for a little boy.

Heroes and villains

From Nanny's house in Aston, we could hear the roar of the crowd on Saturday afternoons and we could see the floodlights and the lamps cleverly arranged in the shapes of the letters 'A' and 'V'. The magic was imprinted on me forever when Dad took me to my first game at Villa Park. I was 7 and cannot remember who we played. I had never seen nor heard such a large crowd of people. Replica kits were still just for kids then, but nearly everyone wore a claret and blue scarf. Giant police horses clopped past. I felt intimidated. Anything could happen. I queued up clutching my fifty pence at a turnstile for juniors. When my turn came, I used all my strength to push through, wondering if I would get trapped forever inside the heavy, clanking mechanism. I emerged into the warm clothing and unfamiliar bodies of the crowd. Although aware that I could not go back through the turnstile and was now moving as part of that crowd, I felt safe somehow. Reunited with my dad, we climbed the seemingly endless steps of the Holte End. I saw lots of boys like me, standing on milk crates or sitting on the metal uprights. It's that electric tingle of shared excitement and belonging I feel every time I go back to Villa Park.

Being a supporter of a football team gives you access to an identity, a sense of belonging to a tribe, and rich family and social traditions. We didn't go to games very often. We spent most weekends looking at houses or, for a few months, caravans. That's to say, my parents looked at the houses and caravans and Anthony and I were usually left to squabble in a hot car. I didn't understand why my parents always seemed to be thinking about their next home. They were surviving in difficult financial times. I didn't know how tough the early-'80s financial recession was. I never noticed because I had everything I needed. We had many happy caravanning holidays in Dorset, and had a fairly reliable family car.

I learned recently that my parents were planning a move to Cornwall, but it never came off. Another pebble in the stream of life that could have profoundly changed my life. Between homes, we lived in a caravan in Oxfordshire for a summer. We had been joined by a new arrival: another brother, Patrick. We had a black-and-white TV that ran off the battery of Dad's van. We all lived together, although I chose to sleep outside in the awning with the dog. One night, there was a commotion inside the van because Anthony had rolled off the top bunk and dropped onto the bed below, badly damaging it. Of course, I had avoided minor injury and a nasty shock, but my unhealthy obsession with Anthony's weight began.

We lived in Minster Lovell, Oxfordshire from 1984. We attended a Church of England school that was only about 100m from where we lived. The greatest difference I noticed was that we didn't have to wear a uniform. The summer holidays seemed endless. I remember playing with friends, but I also spent a lot of time pedalling around the nearby streets on my own. I would catch crickets by sliding a milk bottle down a stalk of grass with a cricket on it, and quickly cover it with my hand – happily thinking the insect would be just as content in a milk bottle with nothing more than a stalk of grass.

My first kiss came on a bright summer's day. I am not too clear as to how it happened. I was wearing my best red T-shirt and trying to get a ball out of someone's garden. I was joined by a girl about my age that I did not know. She wanted to show me how if you ate the flowers on the nettles that grew beside her house, they tasted like sweets. Curious, I followed her. Once we were there, she leaned in for a kiss. It was unexpected, but I just was not interested in girls at that age. I just wanted to ride my bike and play. I don't remember seeing her again.

The '80s and '90s were a rich source of cultural influence. Neither of my parents had been to university and were not consumers of classical art or literature. My dad would get a tabloid paper on Sunday, leaving it to me to discover the power of words outside of the home. We had a bookshelf, weighed down with photo albums and heavy reference books that were never used – just there for appearances. I read everything I could get my hands on at home, mostly instructional books, and the Tolkein volumes my dad had collected in his youth. An eclectic mix. School provided more age-appropriate books, but I was already hooked. I enjoyed the *Adventure* series of Willard Price and the fantasy stories of Enid Blyton, like *The Faraway Tree*.

At Christmas, Uncle Brian would present me with ripping yarns, classics like *Treasure Island*, *The Count of Monte Cristo* and *The Secret Agent*. Gamely trying to expose me to classic literature with limited success. Other adults would play it much safer, giving me book tokens or selecting an exciting film or TV book tie-in for me to read. One such book I remember fondly is *The Box of Delights* (Masefield, 1984). This magical Christmas tale was being shown on TV as I read the book. I remember feeling the exhilaration of reading ahead after each episode and then disappointed that the TV imagining of the book did not come close to my own. The intense feelings of danger and excitement that permeated the story when I read it were missing when I watched it on TV. That was when I realised both TV and books rely on the audience/reader filling in the gaps with their imagination.

I took my copy of *The Neverending Story* (Ende, 1988) to the cinema in 1984 to read along with the film. I wanted to see if films were any better at conveying the magic I felt. The story was about a boy escaping reality into a fantasy world, which he is destined to save. It really appealed to me. You can imagine my disappointment and embarrassment when the film started and the lights went down, making it too dark to read.

I think TV in the '80s was undergoing an identity crisis. Children's TV had innocent and educational stuff like *Rainbow* and *Play School* for the very young. There was still plenty of weird stuff like *Ivor the Engine*, *Mr Benn*, *The Wombles*, *The Magic Roundabout* and *The Banana Splits* still circulating from the '70s. Children's TV soon established regular timeslots on weekday afternoons, but not being sure what kids wanted, broadcasters adopted the same scattergun approach. With a heady mixture of weirdness, the manga-influenced *Battle of the Planets* was shown alongside sitcoms like *Rentaghost*, magazine shows like *Blue Peter*, or dramas like *Grange Hill*. Saturday mornings were peak viewing times for kids, with specially developed shows. I preferred *Swap Shop* to the chaos of *Tiswas*. It was somehow decided that *The Dukes of Hazzard* and *Buck Rogers* were perfectly appropriate for kids watching at Saturday teatimes, and they were exciting and colourful, but watching again as an adult it shocked me how sexually charged they were.

Something that worked well for both kids and adults was *The Muppet Show*. I have no idea who most of the guests were, until Mark Hamill, the actor who played Luke Skywalker in *Star Wars* appeared one night. I loved the silly, colourful, and good-hearted nature of it, where the judgemental voices of Statler and Waldorf were ignored by everyone else. We saw some of the Muppet films at the cinema and I have loved the work of Jim Henson ever since. I think the trick was to provide content for adults and kids, without kids being aware. Think of Pixar's *Up*, a touching story about loss, aging, and regret, which kids see as a story about an old man and his talking dog.

I had a TV in my room, with access to four whole channels, from age 12 and was free to watch as much as I wanted, staying up until the channel finished broadcasting for the night. I was drawn to comedy, such as *Monty Python*, *Blackadder*, *The Young Ones*, *Carry On* films and anything with Norman Wisdom. I eagerly watched most things, especially the edgier output of Channel 4. I appreciated American situation comedies such as *Happy Days*, *Mork & Mindy*, *The Golden Girls*, *Roseanne*, *M*A*S*H**, and *Taxi*. I liked the safety and predictability of the sitcom. No matter what happens to set characters in their set locations, the core dynamic never changes and everything is back to normal by the end, ready for the next episode. They were safe and predictable. Science fiction was also trying to establish itself for adults and kids. Watching TV with my dad in the evenings while Mum was at work, the programmes we watched together (including *Dr Who*, *Star Trek*, *Blake's 7* and *The Day of the Triffids*) had dark, complex, adult storylines and were quite scary. I was challenged and excited rather than traumatised by this. I could not understand why the animated retelling of *The Lord of the Rings* was not for children. After all, it was a cartoon and had frequent singing in it – weren't cartoons supposed to be for kids?

A favourite of mine combined sci-fi, puppetry, and a sitcom: *Alf*. Alf was a loveable, wise-cracking alien, who lived with an '80s American family. Basically, *Happy Days* with an alien instead of The Fonz. Watching *Alf* again recently, I remembered how much I would have loved to have a friend like him. At the time, I was unaware of how gently political the show was (Alf calls the American president to tell him to abandon nuclear weapons), and with his concern for the family finances, I now empathise with the dad of the family.

My dad was far more interested in mainstream film, and our VHS copies of films and TV shows quickly expanded onto our living room shelving. Suddenly, our home was filled with the characters created by Robin Williams, Steve Martin and Gene

Wilder, as well as classics like *Raiders of the Lost Ark*, *Aliens*, *The Goonies* and *Back to the Future* – all the '80s films! Dad was a member of Blockbuster Video and would bring home the latest titles, many meeting his taste for violent action films. His growing VHS collection soon needed its own cataloguing system, with over a hundred cassettes and a book indexing each one.

Star Wars – a fairy tale set in space, full of action and adventure – captured my imagination from an early age. My taste for thrillers, fantasy, and science fiction grew from watching *Flash Gordon*, *Buck Rogers* and *Battlestar Galactica* on TV. Anthony and I used to watch *Star Wars* over and over again; I could replay the entire film in my mind and used to do that to drift off to sleep. We didn't go out very much as a family, so I do remember going to see *The Empire Strikes Back* in the cinema. For some reason, we saw it twice that afternoon. I remember being in awe as we met the Jedi Master, Yoda (essentially a muppet!), and was frightened for most of this very dark film as my heroes were betrayed, frozen in carbonite, or dismembered.

And then it gets even better! Who remembers the dawn of home computers? We were lucky to always have the latest console or computer: from the Atari 2600, through to the ZX Spectrum, Commodore 64, Mega Drives, and PlayStations. I spent hours of my childhood playing them. In the '80s, game graphics were pretty simple and the gameplay basic. A great deal of imagination was required to enjoy them. Usually, the artwork on the front of the box bore no resemblance to the game itself – a good cue for my blossoming imagination. For instance, *Manic Miner*, *Ant Attack*, and *Transylvania Towers*. In this fashion, I was a Grand Prix driver, an overheating security droid, Bruce Lee, a submarine commander or a pilot nursing his B-17 bomber back to base. These games stimulated my brain and provided me with a love of computers that has helped me in adult life. I'm so glad I've been able to continue enjoying this part of my life as my disability progresses.

My Uncle Chris introduced us to the Atari 2600, but I was 10 when basic programming emerged in the mid-'80s. A simple computer language that was accessible to everyone! I was enthralled. And so, my complex and fulfilling relationship with computers began. Dad kept us up-to-date with the computer game scene, getting us magazines with the latest reviews and cheat codes and when he could, the games themselves. A shop selling computer games called Soft Spot opened in Banbury to serve this market. I still like to browse in shops like Game. I would have loved to write creatively on the computer back then, but was limited by being able to print one line at a time on our early printer with its roll of paper. Word processing was seen as serious work, not creative or fun. It wasn't until we had a PC in the '90s that it became possible.

Thank you for the music!

My early years were also full of music. It seemed to be with us everywhere – at home, of course, but also in the car on family journeys. Growing up in the '60s, my parents had fully embraced The Beatles' message of love. They also had fabulous taste in music. My dad liked Neil Diamond, James Taylor, Bob Dylan, Van Morrison, Phil Collins, and Paul Simon. My mum's taste was rooted in The Beatles, although generally more contemporary: The Cars, The Cranberries, Bryan Adams, and Crowded House. Unlike Dad's, it included female artists, such as Blondie, Tracy Chapman, Joan Armatrading, Tina Turner, Kate Bush, the Carpenters, Abba, and Sade. They both liked Led Zeppelin, ELO, Queen, Fleetwood Mac, Tom Petty, David Bowie, Thin Lizzie, and the Eagles. Here's an early acknowledgement to the versatility of audio; my parents also had *The War of the Worlds* musical and Tolkien's *Lord of the Rings* radio play on cassette, but I don't remember them ever listening to the radio.

In our house, loud music was a form of emotional expression and communication. The high volume would signify my mum's feelings of love, or, more usually, displeasure with my dad. It still triggers me if Helen plays a song on repeat to learn it or plays one of her own quite bleak songs. I find myself wondering 'What is she trying to tell me?' My dad played his music at high volume too. I think his immersion in loud music was slightly different; his surrounding himself with beautiful sounds and voices was his way of escaping from a harsh upbringing.

My own appreciation of music began at 11 when I got my first cassette/radio player. I was now able to record chart music from the radio and to play it whatever I wanted. That journey started with loud and rebellious music, even if I didn't understand very much about it. Then, as I grew up, with the influence of my parent's music, I began to appreciate the depth of well-written songs. I was lucky that my parents respected me enough not to criticise my early musical choices and I was able to dip into their extensive music collection as I went.

As an adult, much of my time with music now is spent going much deeper into bands or artists that I love and trust, listening to every song I can, learning about the musicians and their times or going back and exploring the music of my parents. Surrounding myself with the music of my childhood reminds me of that safety and security. When I'm learning more about The Beatles, Elvis, David Bowie or Kurt Cobain (Cross, 2002), I find it so reassuring that they all struggled with how the world saw them. Now my CDs have been boxed up in the loft for a while now, and I stream music from my phone via Bluetooth. I'm listening to broadly the same songs I always have. Wanting to discover fresh new sounds, I stream new music every morning, but rarely find anything that moves me.

I do like all kinds of music, but only good music. I think the secret to good music is a balance between tune, rhythm and lyrics. Lyrics are not essential, they need to be meaningful, clever and/or funny if used, like with rap. I really like music by comedians such as Flight of the Conchords, Tenacious D, Monty Python, and Bill Bailey.

I recently bought my daughter her first CD and MP3 player and added her to our family music subscription. Although I don't play loud music, we do have music in the car and at the dinner table every night. I'm hoping she has heard enough good music from me to begin her own musical journey.

Holy Roman Catholics!

Being a Roman Catholic child made me feel even more special. When Mum married a Catholic, she had to promise that any children would be brought up in the Catholic faith. For some people, this means a lifetime of guilt, fear, and inadequacy. But not me. My dad wasn't super-observant, although he took us to mass every Sunday. I was never particularly aware of being Catholic, or of my Irish descent.

In 1985, we moved to Banbury. A big town with Catholic churches and schools, it meant I could grow up within the Catholic faith. I did not care about the church's teachings. I enjoyed being a pure soul, one of the select few. I knew the rituals, the stories and the correct responses. Unfortunately, I blissfully accepted the outright misogyny, homophobia, and ableism that came with it. I just didn't understand the power of guilt. I remember feeling very confused at my first confession; I couldn't think of any sins I had committed, and had to find things I felt guilty about. With its doctrine of forgiveness, I knew that the Catholic religion was a game that I could play well.

I had a happy few years at Saint John's Primary School in Banbury; although the levels of religious instruction were higher than anything I'd experienced before, I felt secure there. I soon found that a polite, fair-haired boy could do no wrong in a school run by nuns and staffed by women and a single male teacher. One year, the school put on a play of the Easter story and performed it in the town's Catholic church. I was given the part of Judas, and had a few verses to sing solo. Judas is one of the most hated figures in the Bible. Far from being upset, I felt sympathy for him. We're all human, and for no reason he had the hardest test of his soul – one that he was bound to fail. Someone he loved needed him to fail. What if both Jesus and Judas knew this and Judas had to perform the world's most disgusting treachery anyway? Maybe I should have been an actor!

The only time I pushed the boundaries of organised religion was one afternoon after lunch when I claimed to have seen an angel above the playground. Miracles happened all the time and the Catholic teaching promoted it. From the miracles of mass, to the trips to Lourdes that the school organised, God's world was full of wonder. My class had been shown a video about some Romanian children who had been visited by Our Lady. Only the children could hear her voice and they were now famous. It had been recognised by the Pope as a miracle. Why show it to impressionable and imaginative children? Especially one desperate for attention!

So, one clear summer afternoon, when all the children were playing loudly in the playground, the scent of freshly cut grass in the air, I looked up into the sky over the school buildings and, squinting into the sun, saw something hovering up there. A friend was with me and we convinced each other that it was an angel. In reality, it was probably the reflection of the unsteady descent of a tiny dead vein on the surface of my eye. We told our teacher, Sister Jackie, about our angel and I was surprised that we weren't immediately acknowledged as miracle children. Instead, we were sent to different corners of the classroom to 'think about what we had said.'

We moved again in 1987 to Barford St Michael, a small village about 5 miles south of Banbury that Dad had discovered on his way to work in Oxford. My parents wanted to stay in the same area so as not to disturb our education. Also, they had finally found their Shire. My first memory of the village was driving along a single-track road on a sunny spring afternoon, the road lined with blossoming horse chestnut trees.

At about this time, with her children at school, my

mum was starting her own journey of independence. Driving was a key factor, and Mum showed great perseverance by failing her driving test nine times before finally passing. She worked in childcare, eventually as a county council inspector of nursery and homecare facilities. She enjoyed the work and was extremely good at it. Socially, there was little to do in the village, but there were enough people around my age to share growing-up with.

At age 11, I moved to the local Catholic secondary school, only one of two in Oxfordshire. Opened in 1962 and named for a Jesuit priest who was martyred in Oxford in 1610, there were more masses, prayers, and an active paedophile chaplain (convicted in 2012). There were small groups of Italian and some Irish families, and a lot of my classmates were from other religious backgrounds, or none at all. The school had grown, adding a large chapel, but it was still small enough to keep its own identity. I was shocked to find that the roles that I had mastered did not work in that tougher social climate. I was nervous and apprehensive. At the end of the day, I just wanted to do well and please the teachers. Regrettably, I was too open, too vulnerable, and this attracted bullies.

On my first day, I remember someone running past me and knocking my half-eaten sandwich out of my hand. It landed in a puddle. Instantly, I felt tears rise as I looked at its remains and thought of the work that my mum had put into making it for me. Anxiety and guilt choking me with their bony hands, I realised that this reaction was a weakness I could not afford to have. I needed to learn to hide my feelings from *other people*. For the first time, I wondered if I was really as special as everyone seemed to think. Had I lost my childhood superpower?

Besides this intimidation and judgement at school, getting there on the school bus was worse. Now we lived in a village, I relied on the school bus to take me the 6 miles to school. The bus also served another secondary school and a sixth-form college. Our village was the last pick-up on the route, so the bus was packed when it arrived. The village children who I was friends with went on an earlier bus, so the only children catching my bus were children going to that school from villages further out, kids going to the sixth form centre at Banbury School, and those few who attended the same school as me.

I still have dreams about this giant, dirty machine full of my peers pulling up, all watching as I clamber aboard, lurching awkwardly down the crowded aisle littered with bulky holdalls as the bus pulls away, lifting my eyes, reading the body language of anyone with an empty seat next to them, trying not to look desperate, and trying to maintain my composure. Making the right choice here was important. I went through this ordeal twice a day for six years. I don't think I realised at the time how stressful this was. The bus was a microcosm of teenage society; everyone had a definite place based on which friends and relatives also travelled on the bus, and their reputation at school. The older kids slouched at the back, surrounded by smoky mystery.

The bus became an alternative existence for me. I played the game and held my own. My confidence grew, until I was sitting on the back seat. When I got to school each morning (usually a few minutes late), I had to start the whole process over again. Being late for school was pretty usual, and it left me feeling alienated most mornings. It probably didn't help that I chose to take a briefcase to school in my second year.

Another massive trial was catching the bus in the afternoon. For some reason, it picked us up from the neighbouring rival school. The shortest route was over two bleak sports fields that quickly became muddy and waterlogged in the winter. The mud was so thick it could suck your shoes and socks off! If you weren't on the bus when it drove away, you missed it. Before mobile phones, this meant a long and lonely walk home.

I also began to develop friendships and find hobbies. I began going to public speaking events with the school; my favourite topic was: 'Should we use nuclear power?'. It was probably the state school equivalent of debating. I would argue the pros and cons myself. I didn't know that my cousin, Spencer, would become a world champion debater himself. Because it was 1988, and enjoying the company of other nerds, I joined a lunchtime *Dungeons & Dragons*' group.

One teacher saw straight through me – he didn't like what he saw. Bob Taylor was the head of languages. In his 50s, with a crumpled grey suit and short, scruffy, wiry hair, he smoked cigars and ran the school discos. A paternal figure; also someone to share a joke with. We could tease him that his cough sounded bad, cheekily ask why our homework had not been marked on the day we handed it in, or tease that we would report him to Childline for his temper. But there was a line as he had an explosive temper.

My form room was adjacent to his classroom and we often heard explosions from there. *'Zut alors!'* he would curse loudly – as if it either made him French, or we couldn't understand it was a swear word because it was French. Then we would hear slamming doors as he left his bewildered class to burst into ours, crimson with rage, to consult with our teacher, a native French-speaker. While this middle-aged English man vented his rage in broken French, she would have to nod politely and reply in slow, basic French.

I got on the wrong side of him early in my time at school. 'Where is your homework? Where is your exercise book?' he demanded. All the class turned to look at me. I shrugged my shoulders or gave a weak excuse. 'Come up here,' he ordered. I rose and approached slowly, not knowing what was about to happen. When I reached the front, he grabbed my wrist. 'Come with me to the head.' In what was probably a repeat of what an angry teacher had said to him once, he added, 'You are idleness personified!' as he marched me to the head's office. As I waited, I felt like the world was ending. I suppose that was what Mr Taylor wanted. With the head unavailable, and after a long wait, I was buzzed in to see the deputy head. He had a large golden retriever occupying the office with him, which lifted its head as I entered the office. I think Mr Cousins was used to being sent pupils by Mr Taylor, who obviously had challenges in classroom management. I knew that showing how sorry and upset you were seemed to work with grown-ups, so I brushed away a tear and looked at the floor. Realising how upset I was, Mr Cousins gave me the Jesuit (ultra-hard-working Christian) take on the importance of hard work and its rewards in this life and in heaven, and sent me to wait outside the classroom until the lesson ended. In between my class leaving and the next class arriving, I was to collect my bag and coat and apologise to Mr Taylor.

I appreciate now that Mr Taylor was frustrated with me for not realising my potential, and he was one of the few teachers who intervened. He must have seen something in me that reminded him of what he could have done if he'd worked harder at school. After this incident, I felt that I had earned a little respect from my classmates and I always did my homework for Mr Taylor. Bob Taylor was my favourite teacher; he is fondly remembered by many other students too.

As anyone who grew up in the '80s knows, nuclear war was a terrifying and very real threat. My mum had joined the CND (Campaign for Nuclear Disarmament) and was a member of the Banbury branch. I went with her to vigils and protests and made and distributed placards. We went on a 'peace picnic', playing a dramatic game of cat-and-mouse with the police as we looked for somewhere to eat our sandwiches. We stayed at a peace camp on the perimeter of the sprawling US airbase at Upper Heyford to protest against having nuclear weapons in our country. Not owning a tent, we slept in our Volvo Estate with the seats down. Most of the other protesters were women and children – some of them had been at the camp for months. Bruce Kent, the leader of the CND, was leading the march and I remember lying in the road and feeling the greatest camaraderie with the other protesters. I learned that protest is important and began to appreciate, respect, and value the contribution of women.

Dad had always been a drinker; in Barford, he began brewing his own beer, wine, and cider. He would famously mix his home brew in the bath, doubling up on the ingredients for extra strength. Sometimes I would help mix his concoctions with a special spoon; I loved the malty smell that arose when he added the hot water. The airing cupboard and garage stored demijohns of beer or wine in various stages of fermentation. He would drink the beer with meals and for refreshment. I thought nothing of making Mum a cup of tea and filling up Dad's pewter tankard from the barrel in the kitchen and bringing their drinks out together.

My youngest brother, Pat, had the great fortune to be the youngest member of the family. He benefitted from the wisdom my parents had gained from bringing up two boys (no spankings for him!). His happy childhood was derailed by events that were coming to our family. Only 6 himself, he had taken up kung fu at the village hall. A multi-talented and humble friend of my parents called Paul was teaching the classes. I liked the idea of being a martial arts master and the respect it would get me at school and on the school bus, so with a Kung Fu suit and a dragon pole dad fashioned from a broom handle, I joined up. At the same time, my girlfriend, Liz, and her friend, Tracie – who I think had been persuaded into it – joined up too. Too young and poor to frequent the village pub, it was the only kind of social activity to be found in the village that had grown while its amenities had not.

Paul favoured traditional methods of training: hard work, repetition, endurance, and a bit of humiliation. At the end of each lesson, there would be a sparring session with someone of a comparable size. I was usually pitched against Tracie, who would invariably end my participation with a sharp kick to my crotch. Even worse was when we had to spar with Paul himself. Like something out of a '70s martial arts movie, he would have the whole group rush at him one after the other while he blocked and kicked us away. I remember sliding on my back to the edge of the room, getting up, taking a deep breath, and running back for more.

This looks like a job for ...

When I was about 13, I was told about a job available on a chip van belonging to a man in the next village. I enquired and went to meet him. Kevin was a giant of a man, with a friendly demeanour and a farmer's work ethic. He had a giant personality and giant hands to match. The job was every Sunday at Finmere Market and every other Saturday at Milton Keynes Market.

The work was physically and mentally demanding. Large gas cylinders, bins full of uncooked chips, boxes full of burgers, sausages and fishcakes had to be manhandled into and out of the back of a Mercedes van. There were no tills, so every order had to be calculated mentally. The cleaning, food preparation, and tidying up never ended. We wouldn't leave either market until after dark. I didn't have a seat in the van, just a piece of wood spanning the gap between driver and passenger seats. The weather was shocking during the winter. It would be dark and freezing in the mornings. Although the markets weren't busy until nine, we had to get there, set up and be serving the traders with breakfast before eight. Finmere Market was held on a vast airfield where the wind whipped through the open ground. Some mornings we would unpack and find that the vinegar had frozen in its bottles.

On my first day at Milton Keynes, Kevin sent me to borrow a 'long weight' from another trader. I remember getting more and more anxious as I followed its trail from one trader to another. I did not want to let my new boss down on my first day. When I returned an hour later, empty-handed and dejected, he asked with a grin if I had gotten a long wait. He must have had a farmer's sense of humour too.

I worked the job for a couple of years; always paid with a plastic money bag full of pound coins. I learned valuable lessons about not being afraid of hard work and earning my own money. The first thing I bought was a leather jacket and a pair of PONY high-top trainers, wearing both constantly for several years until they fell apart. Soon I had saved enough to buy the electric guitar I craved – seeing this as another icon that could give me the status I was so hungry for.

I was 14 when I decided that smoking would go a long way toward making me the kind of person I wanted to be. Operating on the fringe of society, smokers lurked at the back of the bus shrouded in mystery – and cigarette smoke! Smoking was non-conformist and, as far as I could see, it clearly separated the bullies from the bullied. Mum was a heavy smoker and had been for as long as I could remember, which further normalised it for me. The first packet of cigarettes I bought were from the vending machine in the village pub; sixteen for three shiny 50p pieces. I had chosen my brand based on the popularity of Marlboro with rock bands like Guns N' Roses. I was going to be a glamour smoker. By only smoking at the right times, I was going to use smoking as the social tool that I needed, without getting addicted. I sat on the windowsill in my bedroom and smoked my first cigarette. Not liking the taste and my head spinning so much I almost fell out of the window, I was nevertheless pleased with the image of me holding a cigarette, and the fact that I was changing. I bought cigarettes and smoked them on my breaks on the chip van. A couple of years older than me, my girlfriend at the time also smoked. The smoking group had girls in it too.

February 1991 was my first concert. Now I had money, I could finally afford to go and see the bands I worshipped. I went to see Megadeth at the Birmingham NEC. The support band were grunge pioneers Alice in Chains. I stood near the front and became very worried when a mosh pit opened in front of where I was standing. The fashionable phenomenon where crowds created a gap in front of the stage and people took boundless joy in hurling themselves and others into it. The look of abject terror in my eyes as someone grabbed me to throw me into the whirling pile of bodies was enough to make them let go. Later, I caught a plectrum from Dave Mustaine, my hero. Exhilarated, I came out into the chilly night air to find that I was completely soaked in sweat. I was forever changed. Capable of standing on my own two feet. I went off to meet Dad, who took me in his van to concerts.

I went to see quite a few bands in the '90s, in arenas, smaller venues, and at outdoor festivals. These were the closest I came to a spiritual experience. In the sense of being part of a mass celebration, with a little danger and witnessing breathtaking moments. It was also in a safe environment, surrounded by my people. However, when watching The Cult at Milton Keynes National Bowl in 1993, with the crowd swelling forwards and backwards, I was horrified to find that I couldn't pick my feet up to keep with them and was at risk of going under and being trampled to death. It felt like people several miles away were standing on my untied shoelaces. When that song ended, I managed to extract myself and watched the rest of their set from much further back. I rejoined the crowd later that day, shoelaces firmly tied and the ends tucked into my shoes, to watch Guns N' Roses play a brilliant set. An unforgettable, almost spiritual moment for me was during an Aerosmith concert at Monsters of Rock in 1994, when a low-flying jet buzzed the stage with perfect timing during 'Living on the Edge.'

The electric guitar I bought was a black Fender Squier Stratocaster with a white scratch plate and a maple neck. I had saved up from my job on the chip van and Dad and I went to Milton Keynes on my birthday to get it. A neighbour lent me a Marshall Bluesbreaker amplifier. Soon after, I bought an effects pedal. I gave learning the guitar a fair try. To be honest, I was always more interested in how I looked with the guitar, rather than how I sounded. I spent a lot of my practice time playing along to rock music I had recorded from my parents, or from my own small collection of vinyl and on my cassette player. In a nod to image, I later traded the guitar for a denim jacket with music patches sewn around it and a chain hanging from the back. To me it was well worth it, just for the feeling of self-assurance that the jacket gave me while I was wearing it. The guitar later turned up with the guitarist in *Clarion*, a local band. I am proud to say that Billy has been having guitar lessons since he was 8 and shows great promise of being the great guitarist I never was.

In an expression of rebellion and frustration, I took my parents' car after closing time one night and decided to drive it home from the pub at the other end of the village. I started the engine and felt adrenalin surge through me. I then realised that, like playing the guitar, I didn't know how to make the thing work. I didn't know which pedal did what, or how to change gear, but I wasn't going to be deterred by a lack of knowledge. I rifled through the glovebox and flipped through the manual. I put the car in first and pulled away. I didn't change gear again. I was steering for my life, with the engine screaming and a smell of burning oil in my nostrils. I negotiated a long row of parked cars and took the sharp left bend by the church. This hairpin bend also has a steep gradient and is bordered on one side by the church's sloping path. I understeered on the sharp corner and hit the side. Terrified, I rolled back and tried again. This time I oversteered and hit the other side, going a considerable way up the steep bank. The car rolled down again and I eventually negotiated the corner at the third attempt. I drove along another narrow street, avoiding more parked cars, and turned into our street with the indicator flashing. I rolled the car in front of the house and turned everything off. Smoke was hissing and hot metal trickled from under the bonnet as I went into our house.

My parents were still up with some friends. I pulled the youngest and most carefree, Marilyn, outside and showed her the damage. A neighbour of ours, nearer my own age and with no kids of her own, I hoped she could help. She told me to go to bed and that she would break the news to my parents. I expected a confrontation that night, but none came. The next morning, I came down and sheepishly awaited their reaction. Choosing to express themselves through music, my parents repeatedly played 'Bat Out of Hell' by Meatloaf. I had to pay towards the repairs from my job for the next few months. In hindsight, I was very lucky that I hadn't killed myself, someone else, or damaged something. I don't know what she said to them – it must have been good.

To make matters worse, the landlady's young son, Spencer, found broken headlight glass on the road by the church, and tyre tracks up the bank on the other side. Putting two and two together, he assumed that one of my parents had hit the wall and came to gloat. He was from Birmingham too, but as a Birmingham City fan (or Bluenose), he relished in the misfortune of Villa supporters. He was quickly told the truth. After that, everyone knew and the way my parents had dealt with it was the best part of the story.

Girls had started to become important to me and, unbeknown to me, I had achieved an acceptable balance between being edgy and nice. Girls of both descriptions were interested in me. I was just not experienced enough to enjoy it. The two girlfriends I had up to the age of 15 were a couple of years older than me. By then, I'd had many short relationships with girls around my age. I took the whole thing far too seriously, and my need for attention, and a jealous frenzy of insecurity, destroyed most of my relationships. I think most of the girls who I went out with must have found me hard work and felt disappointed when they got to know me properly.

Some lived in our village, but not being Catholic like me, they went to a different school. Communication during the day was by letters passed through our mutual friend, Tracie, for whom I secretly yearned, but was always the 'safe' friend. My untidy handwriting had always been an embarrassment to me, so I typed epic letters to my girlfriends on my mum's electric typewriter. Occasionally I'd be moved to write a poem, but many of those letters must have been very complicated!

Then everything changed. Forever.

DIAGNOSIS

Before *You've Been Framed* was on British TV, Dad filmed me falling flat on my face on the beach. As the sea shrank back, I staggered and fell over. One for the family archive!

The previous section gives you an idea of the me growing up – my influences and experiences and the kind of person I was becoming. I was a bright, happy person with a conviction of my own specialness. My earliest recollection of anything wrong with my balance was that instance on the beach as a child, with the clear water breaking over my feet. As the sea retreated, it felt as if the floor had disappeared. I lost my balance and fell. In my last year at primary school, I would often sprain my ankle in the playground. As I grew, my clumsiness and poor balance often came out in sports. By 14, I could not sprint and stay in the same lane. Once I crumpled in a heap after about three-quarters of the 100m. I had to jog or walk on cross-country runs, finishing exhausted and last. My friends and PE teachers were as mystified as I was. I thought it was a growth problem, which would right itself when my brain caught up with my body. I tended to enjoy sports that didn't involve running, playing in goal, and field events.

There were also signs present in my job on the chip van. I could not carry cups of boiling tea or coffee – even with a lid on. My slow, concentrated walk across the floor of the van was too much. I still smile to think of the horrified look on my colleagues' faces as I threw cups of scalding liquid all over the place. Pretty soon, hot drinks were no longer my responsibility!

I was finally referred to a nearby hospital for tests. As it was a few years before Ataxia UK backed the work to identify many neurological conditions through a blood test, I was subjected to having electrical impulses passed through my nerves in my arms, hands, legs and feet over a couple of days, to observe my muscle reaction. If you've ever felt a slightly unpleasant electrical current put your hair on end, or give you a static shock, you can imagine a more intensified surge pulsing through your limbs, making them jerk painfully and unrecognisably. I felt like I was being unfairly punished for something. A few months later, my parents were called to our GP's office and were given the grim news. I had been diagnosed with Friedreich's ataxia. An inherited neurological condition. It is progressive and, as yet, incurable. The news was that I would be lucky to survive into my mid-thirties, at which point I would have lost control over my body and only be able to carry out automatic functions – blinking, breathing, and swallowing. To add to this, I would also have a high chance of developing commonly associated complications along the way: diabetes, heart problems, curvature of the spine and feet – oh, and loss of vision and hearing.

This shattering news was accompanied by paralysing fear, anger, deep denial, and guilt. I felt alone. I'm sure we all did. I felt guilt for letting my parents down and anger at them for passing this down to me. They not only felt helpless but were wracked with guilt themselves. Without counselling or support, we all fell apart. Broken-hearted, Dad's heavy drinking spiralled out of control. Mum had to rely on others for support. I felt we were all shaken so much by the diagnosis that we had to rebuild our lives and ourselves. It equalised my parents and I, blurred the distinction between child and adult, which no teenager needs. My younger brother inherited the diagnosis from me by proxy. Fraternal antagonism between us became merciless bullying on my part. Desperate to protect their remaining son, my parents gently steered my youngest brother away from a formal diagnosis, even though he did not exhibit any signs. I think this impossible choice caused as many problems for him as knowing for sure.

I received a handwritten, heartfelt letter from my Godfather, Uncle Ken, genuinely expressing his great sorrow. I really thought grief was the only way of looking at my situation. Because of his Irish roots, he understood disability in terms of tragedy, sickness and shame. Consumed by grief, I threatened to kill myself before needing to use a wheelchair. What a painful statement for my parents to have to deal with.

My dad did what he could to make things better; he turned to the powerful institutions in his life, trying the Catholic Church first. Social ideology has shifted since then. With its persisting medieval attitudes, the Catholic Church, at least in our experience, was no help. It saw disability as God's punishment, which could only be cured by a miracle or prayer. Unfortunately, such interventions had to be paid for. Dad's idea was to have prayers said for his sons at Lourdes, a place of pilgrimage due to the apparitions of Our Lady. The parish often organised pilgrimages there because they view it as a powerful and holy place in France where sick people can be healed. The monsignor agreed, but explained that two donations would be required. One for the shrine itself, the other for the priest who would be saying the prayers. Dad remembers, 'He didn't want to know how we were, he just wanted to make sure that the donations were clearly marked.'

Undeterred, Dad reached out to another institution that profoundly affected our lives – football clubs. He wrote to Aston Villa and Liverpool (Anthony's team) on behalf of his sons and received match tickets for his trouble. At least the football clubs were there for him.

A neighbour also worked for British Airways and was able to find an opportunity for my dad to courier a package to Paris. As a treat, he took me with him. Shortly after take-off, in the glorious days before high-level security, I was invited into the cockpit. In a beautiful moment I will always remember, we broke through the morning clouds into the clear blue sky, the sun shining brightly. I had to shield my eyes from the light. It had been overcast and rainy that morning. Perhaps that is a nice metaphor for something!

We had an enjoyable day in Paris: climbing the Eiffel Tower, looking around the Notre-Dame Cathedral, and almost getting run over by the most aggressive traffic I had ever seen at the Arc de Triomphe. When it was time to get the bus back to the airport, the driver wouldn't let us on because our tickets were singles, not returns. We had just bought a chalk portrait of me from a street artist with the last of our money, so the driver held his hands in the most Gallic way possible, and we got off. The bus pulled away without us – I *really* hate missing buses.

It was the early '90s and cash was still king, so I sold the only thing of value I had on me: a nice chrome Zippo lighter. An American tourist waiting at the bus stop gave us ten Francs for it – enough to pay for two single coach tickets to the airport. Unfortunately, we had missed our flight back to where Dad had parked in Birmingham, but we managed to get seats on the last commuter flight back to Heathrow. We had certainly had an adventure. Within the panic of us both being lost in a foreign country, I felt the balance shift between my dad and I, with me taking more of the initiative.

Like my parents, I also searched for wisdom following my diagnosis. As a classic 'wounded healer' himself, John Lennon seemed to have plenty. 'Crippled Inside' from his 1971 album, *Imagine*, is a song that really spoke to me. In this upbeat country and western number, Lennon croons in a cheerful southern drawl. It's a bleak stab at the hypocrisy in our society of judging others on appearance alone. It is well known that his 'bizarre obsession for cripples, spastics, any human deformities and people on crutches […] was a subject which was to manifest itself throughout John Lennon's years of fame.' (Coleman, 1995, p. 86)

Listening as a teenager struggling to come to terms with his own disability some twenty-five years after it had been written helped me to begin to understand my condition in a new way. I explained that if people can look fine on the outside and be 'crippled' inside, the reverse must be true. Others will judge you on your physical appearance. Your appearance doesn't make you who you are; don't let others judge you. It just took me a few years to realise this.

Life was difficult after this terrible, life-changing diagnosis, but I felt OK physically. Mentally, I was in trouble; I felt crippled inside. Much like a prisoner facing a death sentence or a soldier trying to survive with death all around, I lived a 'provisional existence', with no aims or goals. Convinced I had no future, I felt I didn't have to take any responsibility for my actions. Deep down, I knew a terrible future awaited me. I became an early edgelord. A dramatic rule-breaker and attention seeker. In today's sense, an edgelord is an individual who uses the Internet to post provocative opinions, such as nihilism or extremist views, in an attempt to impress or shock others. My GCSE year was fast approaching; unfortunately I had already given up on schoolwork. Speaking to people around me at school years later, they all remembered there was something dramatic happening to me, yet weren't sure what it was.

Dissident

My diagnosis destroyed my inner belief that I was special in some way and had an enormous effect on myself and my family. My childhood superpower had gone, but I was still a teenager, and now carrying a shameful secret. I was very confused.

A bright spot for me in those years was the village pub, the George Inn. It quickly became the centre of my universe. I met Helen there, and later her dad started to join us for late-night curries. My parents were popular regulars. Spencer, the son of the landlady, and only a few years older than me, was taking more of a role in running the pub. Using his passion for live music, he started the pub's popular live music nights. He reframed the George Inn and attracted a younger clientele; mainly university students who lived in nearby villages and were all a few years older than me. They were all heroes to me. Especially Dan, a big, friendly chap with a passion for music, who was like a big brother.

Amongst some of the people that Mum talked about were the younger regulars, Clive and Paul and their sisters, and what nice people they were in particular. The first time I met them was when they were playing a very drunken game of pool – I think they were celebrating Clive's birthday. They were both witty and creative young men, who had picked up a lot more life experience than I had. We shared a love of surreal comedy and could quote at will from *Monty Python*, *Withnail and I*, *The Young Ones* or *Blackadder*. I joined their friendship group, who had been engaging in role-playing adventures since their schooldays.

I knew from school that role-play games are a safe way to explore emotions, forget yours, and adapt to unexpected situations. All in a safe environment. Twice a week, we would play. I love laughing and making people laugh; I can laugh hysterically sometimes. When Gary, a gifted artist, rejoined the group a few years later, he would quickly sketch observations that would make me laugh so much that I had to wait for my tea to cool and make sure that Gary and, later, his brother, Martin, were paying attention to the game so I could drink my tea in safety!

Socialising is an important aspect of role-playing too. We had Christmas parties with awards for the best death, best player-character, etc. I recently found a home-made Top Trumps game with thirty-six laminated cards of a baffling array of things that we found funny, many from the worlds of sci-fi, kids' TV, animals, and popular culture. My characters would often have a flaw or difficulty of some kind, which made them fun to play. They were outsiders like me. The most memorable were: Jack O' Diamonds, a charming, thoroughly ruthless rogue; Marco and Amy, the resourceful street-urchin twins; Sir Lionel of Rowe, a gay knight with his best years behind him and no one to settle down with; and Heb, smooth-headed, unlikeable, and violently bad-tempered priest of the moon. Gary would draw portraits of our characters, making them even more real.

Some of the members of the folk band Fairport Convention lived in the village and their annual reunion festival was held in the nearby village of Cropredy. Although I didn't care much for folk music, the custom of camping out at a music festival with my music-loving friends was fantastic. We would all pitch our tents together to form a tented village. This group grew to include younger people from the community and combined nicely with our *Dungeons & Dragons* group to form a perfect storm. Those never-ending teenage summers were some of the happiest of my life.

Spencer shared an interest in medieval history with Clive and Paul, and as they were both professional artists they came up with producing an epic portrayal of the Battle of Agincourt. The difference was that a dozen or so of the figures were to be given the faces of pub regulars. I was to be a young English knight and went to their office in Banbury to have polaroids taken of me wielding an imaginary sword. The story was picked up by local media and we were interviewed by a TV news crew. When asked why I had taken part, I answered, 'I am hoping to impress more women!' With hindsight, I'm glad I said the words 'more' and 'women', but of course the painting did nothing of the kind, and my comments were cut from the final broadcast.

Unable to drive myself, and with no public transport to speak of, and when my parents couldn't, I began regularly hitching the 5 miles between Banbury and home wearing a black raincoat and listening to my Walkman in all weathers. I stood on the corner of Woodworm Studio's lawn at the edge of the village and stuck my thumb out. I was lucky that I had no bad experiences, and was often picked up by people that knew me from the village, including Helen's mum. I was drawn to the quiet village churchyard. In the summer months, when the grass around the church was short, I would lie on the warm earth for hours sometimes, listening to the birds, the wind in the trees, and watching the clouds drift by. Often, my thoughts would linger on the granite war memorial. I would wonder who the dozen names belonged to, what kind of men they were and how they died. I did not recognise any of the eleven names on it from the local families I knew.

It may have been a form of escape; being around such a solemn place surrounded by the beauty of nature and with no possibility of being disturbed really appealed to me and is something I miss. I have always been able to 'tune out' and just drift away. I think sound, or no sound, may be the key to why I liked it so much as this place mirrored the seasons or time of day at which you visited. During the winter, it was cold, wet, and unwelcoming. The crunching gravel path seemed to merge with the squelching mud and fallen leaves. At dusk, the bats would flutter around the Norman porch in their erratic flight. At night, the churchyard was sinister and dark. The musty smell of graveyard dew seemed to be much stronger, the rustling wind sounded louder. But somehow, I knew the occupants of the graves were not malevolent, they were villagers just like me.

McRobin Hood

I started work at McDonald's in Banbury just after my 16th birthday. My experience on the chip van stood me in good stead for the expected hard work. Initially I only worked on busy Saturdays, because of my school commitments. It acted as an escape from my forthcoming GCSEs that I was unprepared for. I quickly made friends with the staff and managers alike. I missed many of my exams; for some subjects with a coursework element, there was little point even sitting them.. I passed English and French with good grades. I think these were my stronger subjects because my teachers encouraged me.

Just after exams were over, the first physical diversion from the life I wanted presented itself. Instead of going to sixth form with my friends, I went full-time at McDonald's. I took it seriously and soon became a reliable, hard-working member of the team. I gravitated toward the customer-facing and organisational jobs. On Saturdays I would work 'backroom', which consisted of making sure that everything was cleaned from breakfast, and that no one in the entire store ever ran out of anything: tartar sauce, clean cloths, lettuce, burger boxes, cups, lids, fries, ice, frozen burgers, napkins – you get the idea. After the lunchtime rush, I would bring down all the stock needed for the evening, and put frozen deliveries away in the giant walk-in freezer, always being sure to carefully rotate the stock. (To this day, I still insist on putting our chilled shopping away!) I was reliable and worked hard. This job involved constant movement and forward planning, and I made it my own. I regularly won employee of the day awards on busy Saturdays and was responsible for training new staff. I picked up the nickname 'Charlie' because of the surname 'Brown' and had it printed on my badge. I soon earned all six stars! The press-on stars were awarded to show proficiency in all the areas of the restaurant, but did not come with an increase in pay or authority. Physically, I was able to carry out my duties in this noisy and busy environment and enjoyed this job because it was a chance to get away from under the shadow of the diagnosis and everyone who wanted to help me.

Occasionally, I would show a group of birthday party kids the walk-in fridge and freezer. I would let a few brave volunteers go inside, only to shut the door and turn the lights off. Delighted screams would ensue and I would open the door again. Once, to my horror, the door sealed itself and it took me a few attempts to open it. The brave adventurers emerged, smiling, and with a great story, completely oblivious to my panic.

There was only one changing room, with a bank of lockers at one end and tables for staff to sit at whilst on a break. Most of the employees came into work already wearing their uniform. It always surprised me that some of the female employees thought nothing of standing in their underwear and using the iron to press their clothes in front of their colleagues. I liked a female co-worker who was a little bit older than me and needed a friend. Bubbly and chatty, I think she got on most people's nerves, but we got on, and we soon became closer. People would tease us whenever we worked the same shifts together because we chatted so much. At one company social event, we enjoyed a slow dance together and the tension between us grew. We sat together on the bus on the way home and, in a confused ten minutes, I told her about my diagnosis, she cried, and then we kissed passionately. We spent the rest of the journey in each other's arms.

After eighteen months, I was sacked from this job I loved for gross misconduct. The kitchen relied on the judgement of a manager looking out over the queues and instructing the kitchen to produce food to their orders. It was better to overproduce and this frequently happened. Any excess food was thrown away, carefully counted, and rendered inedible before being disposed of in the skip outside. It was difficult to see the value of a product when you put so much effort into producing it, and then into destroying some of it. The incident that got me sacked was mostly to do with my poor judgement. A couple of people I knew from school came in. I produced their order for the price of a cup of tea, and they went away. Having just finished my shift, I was called to the counter some minutes later. One friend I had served was throwing his food about and causing some disturbance. The manager wanted to look at the orders on my till to see if he had paid to eat in the restaurant. Unable to find the order on my till, and as nobody in the previous hour had ordered the same items, it didn't look good for me. I protested my innocence and was suspended without pay pending a disciplinary hearing.

Of course, I enjoyed the thrill of breaking the rules and the gratitude of my friends. For a long time, I maintained that the main reasons for my 'generosity' were my rebellious 'Robin Hood' spirit and the chronic wastage of the food that remained unsold after a certain length of time. But I wonder how much I was influenced by my dad's 'adversarial' work-ethic that you should always put yourself before your greedy employer. The hearing was a formal affair held a week later in the small office upstairs. The managers asked if I knew the customers, to which I replied, 'Yes.' I continued to deny giving them free food. The managers concluded that I had been caught. Seeing no point in arguing further, I accepted their verdict and immediate dismissal perhaps too readily. As I left to clean out my locker, the senior manager said, 'I thought you were one of the good guys.' I just shrugged and turned away, ashamed.

The phrase in French *'Avoir l'esprit de l'escalier'* means to think of a witty comeback on the way out of a situation; I wish I had said that I *was* one of the good guys because I didn't accept McDonald's company 'ethics' and relied on my own moral code. Oh well, *c'est la vie*.

An ordinary everyday teenager

Although not making any significant progress, I was pleased that my life revolved happily around casual work, women, and socialising. After a few months without a job, a friend in the village told me about a junior position available at a local bike shop at which he worked. The job involved basic cycle repair, as well as sales work. My friend took me to Banbury in his lovingly restored Triumph Spitfire every day. The shop owner, himself nearing retirement, was unconvinced that I could work for him due to my disability. The only signs of disability I exhibited at that time was that I was slightly unsteady on my feet; it must have been barely noticeable. The only problem was that the new bikes were stored above the shop and carrying a mountain bike packed in cardboard up or down this wide staircase whilst clinging precariously onto the banister was the only thing I found difficult. I had to ask someone else to do this. Initially taken on for a single-month trial, it was extended to a second month to cover the holiday of the manager. Again, I worked hard and was always punctual; I got on well with the other employees and did what I was told.

Once again, romance blossomed. Whilst working in the shop, I had noticed a pretty, delicate-looking girl with an olive-green army coat and a sand-coloured army rucksack walk past the window twice a day. After a few days, I plucked up the courage to wave and smile, and she waved and smiled back. One Saturday afternoon, I saw her in the street and rushed outside to talk to her. I managed to find out that she was studying at the local college, and that she was single. I also managed to get her phone number. Our first date was at the cinema, where we spent most of the film kissing passionately. Her family were all very nice people, and I liked them. We were an item for a few months before I became aware that she was also having problems coming to terms with my diagnosis. We both allowed our relationship to slip away.

The bike shop let me go after Christmas too. The old-fashioned owner had been uncomfortable with my diagnosis as well. These events gave me my first experience of how others' perceptions of disability could affect my future. I lost direction at this point and resigned myself to a future without many of the things I wanted. The self-image that I had nurtured for so long faced a massive complication, disability, and a painful image, a wheelchair.

In 1994, I was with Clive and Paul after an evening down the pub when I found out that Kurt Cobain had died. I had tickets to see Nirvana at the Aston Villa Leisure Centre that March, and I really felt everything was building to that moment. I was finally going to meet my hero and we were going to be as one. Unfortunately, Kurt Cobain overdosed earlier in the tour and the show was cancelled. He was found dead at his home in Seattle a month later. For many, the death of Lady Di in 1997 was the most significant death of the decade, but for me, and many who grew up in the '90s, Kurt Cobain's loss was. I really admired his energy. A fellow nihilist, he had shown the greatest resilience to get what he thought he wanted. In the end, he was so badly damaged that his hard-won fame destroyed him.

Saddened by his death, the pictures of teenagers holding candlelit vigils took me back to the killing of John Lennon in 1980, and I understood what my parents had felt at the loss of one of their heroes. He, too, exuded power and unashamed vulnerability – another 'wounded healer'. For comfort, I immersed myself in the emerging conspiracy theories that Kurt did not choose to leave his fans but was murdered. Cobain's untimely death further convinced me that my own life was worthless and that ending it was a reasonable solution to problems I would face in the future. I know I caused great distress to people when I spoke about my conviction to take my own life before I had to use a wheelchair.

In the meantime, I decided to get a tattoo. This was at a time when getting inked was a subculture, and frowned on by the mainstream. I knew people that were into body art, and of course there had been tattoos in rock music for years. I wanted to be taken seriously. I eventually went to a tattoo parlour in Banbury with my idea. I wanted something ugly and dramatic to remind me that my body held an ugly and dramatic secret that would be with me forever. I chose a strand of black barbed wire to loop around my upper arm. Of course, my decision was as much to do with making a considered fashion statement. (This was several years before Pamela Anderson made the design famous in the 1996 film, Barbed Wire!) The pain was a lot less than I thought it would be, and I went home with a bandage over it, eager to show it off to friends.

I was seeing a girl from the next village. Just 16, she had long brown hair, big brown eyes, Mediterranean skin, and a striking, curvy figure. From very early on in the relationship, it was established that I was to, at all costs, avoid her mother, a solicitor, who had been separated from my girlfriend's father for some years. I think her mother would not have approved of her daughter seeing someone with no future – perhaps that was very much part of my attraction for her daughter. I suppose there were three of us in the relationship. Despite never having had the chance to meet her, her daughter and I were together every day that summer. Even now, I occasionally dream about winning over this woman, who would have hated me, and that I went to so much trouble to avoid, but in whose house I spent so much time.

Returning to have my tattoo completed, I had a heart with my girlfriend's name written on a scroll across it. It was a completely foolish impulse and I finally had it removed 25 years later. Our relationship was very good for 18 months, but as usual my insecurity strained it and brought about a gradual breakdown. Eventually, I found out that she had been cheating on me with someone I knew. Although my behaviour was partly responsible, my worst suspicions were confirmed and I took the news very hard indeed.

CONCLUSION: REAL GONE KID

I had a happy and loving childhood, and exciting early teenage years. My parents were in love with each other and loved me very much. I was a very special child to be positioned somewhere between spoilt and privileged. Not spoiled by wealth, but by attention. That feeling of entitlement from my childhood gave me a sense of being destined for greatness and the beginnings of the stubborn resilience that comes with that. I believed that I could be whatever I wanted when I grew up because I possessed qualities that would guarantee my success with ease. Being the first grandchild, first son, escaping Birmingham and going to a Catholic school just confirmed how special I was.

Soon, I realised that my family believed this too and it seemed to be apparent to anyone else I met. Teachers, babysitters, and other kids' parents agreed

Conclusion: Real Gone Kid

what a well-behaved and polite child I was. I was seldom told off, and the rare occasions that an adult admonished me, I felt outraged and hurt, close to tears, and was sure that my parents would feel the same. This didn't do me any damage, yet it left me with a huge need for attention and an unrealistic expectation to try and live up to. Very occasionally, adults would see through this mask. My parents' ideas of gender roles, work, and success, which they had inherited from their parents, were things that influenced me too.

Apart from a visit to the Doctor Who Museum, our family never went to galleries, museums, the theatre or exhibitions and never had family discussions about politics, art or film, as I imagined my well-to-do cousins did. Popular culture and the latest technology were much more important to my dad. He would rather take us to the cinema or watch a video at home. I wondered for a long time if I had missed out somehow, but through remembering the music I heard and the films and TV I watched during my childhood, I realised that great art was actually all around us. By watching a film or TV together or playing music often and loudly, my parents were also sharing their love of art with me. After all, it was the medium they knew best. They taught me how to listen to music. My dad's video collection, although it was quite mainstream, was quite a good collection in the days before online content providers. Thanks to them both, I have a lifelong love of music, film, TV, and computer gaming. This has helped me adapt to the digital world.

Counselling for me and my family would have helped a lot. It's not right to give parents a difficult diagnosis and expect them to pass it on to their children without any support. My diagnosis was a massive implosion that shook us to the core. I felt like everything had been taken away, that all the things I thought my future held for me were gone. It felt like knowing that your lovely home was going to get burgled repeatedly in the future, and there is nothing you can do to stop it. Receiving a diagnosis such as Friedreich's ataxia, and the implications you're told it will have on your life, can take a long time to come back from, and it did set me back years. Any diagnosis doesn't only affect the individual with ataxia themselves, but also their parents and siblings and other family members too. The entire family need ongoing support, initially to process the diagnosis and the associated thoughts and emotions, but then to live with it too.

I was far from being a superhero. I had lost my childhood superpowers, had not found my special abilities or begun to fight for others. No matter how hard I tried, I felt I was drifting further away from the person I wanted to be. I was obsessed with how *other people* saw me. I didn't finish school and began to drift through life. I had given up on me. Thankfully, my parents hadn't. My ataxia wasn't very noticeable yet and I was still living at home and able to enjoy much of being a teenager. Earning a little money, socialising, finding my place in the world, and listening to music. I was drifting, yet I wasn't going anywhere.

Then, at the end of 1995, something happened that was to change my life forever.

Part Two

Rise

It was 1995; I was 19, unemployed, and depressed. I had left school 3 years before with the 3 GCSEs I had actually turned up for. I had no hope, no dreams, and no future. Then I met my future wife, Helen, and her family.

A GIRL FROM MARS

We had both grown up in Barford, a remote Oxfordshire village, but with three and a half years between us, we had never met. We got talking in the George Inn on a Monday music night, and I invited her back to my house to 'see my puppy' – a lively Jack Russell Terrier cross called Dusty. Helen is beautiful and sharply intelligent; she's quiet with an unpredictable streak of fierce determination beneath. She is patient, kind, and has always been amazing to me. Helen is not generally led by emotions, her approach to life tends to be more practical and focused on the moment. She suspects that this may be part of her autism, and it was exactly what someone waiting for a terrifying prognosis to become manifest needed. We connected through the music we loved, and didn't talk about my condition. I just wanted to live in the moment and it wasn't a problem for us yet. This worked for us both – it set me free, and it also gave Helen some emotional support without committing to a future with anyone.

Helen was about to sit her GCSEs and was expected to do well. Straight away, Helen set a clear ground rule: 'My work always comes first,' she warned sternly. I thought her statement was a forceful counter to my oblique nihilism. On reflection, it was more from a very deep fear of letting her parents down. I happily helped with her revision, typing up her notes, and testing her command of Soviet History. I like to think she saw something in me, that she recognised my affinity for history, and encouraged me to develop myself. When I met her parents, I could see where she got it from. They came from the North-East, both went to Oxford University, and had always worked in the public sector. As Socialists, they believe in opportunity for all, and have a strong sense of fairness. Kind and generous people. Susan, an exceptionally bright person, got her Protestant work ethic from her very aspiring family. John, also very bright, had a Catholic upbringing, a loving family, and exceptional teachers. They went to Oxford when education was still free: Susan excelling in law, John falling into teaching.

A favourite Christmas of mine was the one I spent staying at John's mam's house in Darlington, learning about the people, places, and customs of John and Susan's youth. Much of their lives could have been taken from the surreal adventures of the popular northern comedy duo, Vic and Bob! Mine and Helen's early first dates were often with John as neither of us could drive. Aston Villa had just won the league cup again and as a lifelong Arsenal supporter, we bonded over football. Arsenal became my second team and we went to every Villa v Arsenal game for many seasons. I remember Helen sitting stoically beside me through many bitterly cold afternoons. I had had a prescription for glasses since I was about 10, but refused to wear them of course. John, a glasses wearer himself, showed me that wearing glasses was OK.

While their family pushed me to do more, I was finding the Christie family dynamic equally challenging! The extremes of highs and lows, the sheer anxiety, emotions, and arguments – I have never seen anything like it and found it quite intimidating. There was no drama, no sulking, no lengthy silences, and loud music. The slamming doors were provided by Helen's younger sister, but there was certainly no passive aggression. Their attitude to alcohol was far more relaxed. It took me some getting used to. I find it difficult to stop drinking once I start, so some of the drunkest moments I have had have been on Christie family holidays. Everyone was expected to express exactly how they felt at the height of their anger and then apologise after. They welcomed me on a family holiday to Bordeaux in 1998. We had a good time; it was the first time I had been away with them. I remember feeling totally overwhelmed by all of the volatile emotions flying about and wanting to come home again. I am grateful that Helen takes this 'wear your heart on your sleeve' approach, not bottling things up and overthinking things like I do. The Christie family dynamic was by no means ideal, but it was different enough from my own upbringing for me to function well alongside Helen.

Another challenging side to this family life for me was sharing. One evening, we'd ordered a takeaway and I had studied the menu carefully and specified exactly what I wanted. When the meal arrived, we sat down around the dining table without cloth napkins. I was further horrified as people were trying each other's food. 'Ooh, John's got some lovely sauce, Neville!' was cooed in a high-pitched Terry Jones-style voice, as John's plate got passed up the table, large spoons dipping into it on the way. This contrasted with the formal teas I had known in Lichfield. There, you would carefully construct your plate with what you would eat and you couldn't start on the cakes until all the sandwiches were all gone. This was chaos by comparison; this warmth and humility were going to take me some time to get used to!

As a new couple, we immersed ourselves in '90s culture by going to the cinema, concerts, plays, and recordings of some TV shows. *TFI Friday* and *This Morning With Richard Not Judy* (*TMWRNJ*) in 1999. *TMWRNJ* was a double-act sketch show also on BBC2 with Richard Herring playing the impulsive adolescent to Stewart Lee's intellectual parent. It was edgy and funny, with characters and sketches I still think about today. Not using a wheelchair then, but still pretty unstable on my feet, the three of us got to sit on the sofas in front of the audience on the stage floor.

A few minutes before the recording started, Richard came onto the set wearing the head of a giant chicken and holding a tennis racket. 'Who am I?' he asked, swinging his racket in a slow back-hand motion. It was quite a risk. There was an awkward silence and Richard gamely did some more tennis moves to prompt us. I desperately wanted to help. Wimbledon was in full-swing that week, so I started there. After another couple of seconds of agonising silence, I realised it was down to me and blurted out: 'Tim Henman?'

A huge wave of relief. The audience laughed, relieved that they were no longer on the spot. Richard beamed with relief that his joke had landed and I was relieved that I had gotten the answer right in front of my peers and a hero of mine. 'He's a very clever man,' he said to the audience. As he passed, he looked me in the eye and repeated, 'You're a very clever man.' I've told that story a lot over the last twenty years, and am sure I have embellished it, but that's how I remember meeting Richard Herring. You can ask Helen – she was there too!

Despite the pool of people who remember this show seeming to get smaller each year, this turned out to be one of my best ever interactions with a celebrity. We saw Richard Herring at the Edinburgh Fringe and several local venues – I also listen to his excellent RHLST podcast. We still see Stewart Lee whenever he is in Oxford. Re-watching the episode on YouTube reveals how smart Richard actually was.

As music was something we shared, Helen and I saw a lot of bands at venues big and small. Our favourite was The Smashing Pumpkins, who we saw whenever we could. Oxford really provided a link to '90s culture. I really enjoyed *Bottom Live* shows, the frenetic and breathless performances of Rik Mayall and Ade Edmondson, plus being amazed by Derren Brown's incredible mentalist shows. We saw Harry Hill a few times. After one performance in Oxford, I asked him to christen the Stouffer hand puppet we had just bought. Without a pause, he put the puppet on one hand and held the other hand above in a mock blessing. 'I baptise you Stouffer,' he declared in an authoritative voice, making a sign of the cross with his puppet hand.

With much encouragement and support, I signed up for an arts foundation course with the Open University, studying European humanities. I got the books, recorded the TV programmes, and sent my assignments by post. Helen and her mother took me to my monthly tutorials. I really enjoyed the Open University way of learning, with a little bit of everything from the period being studied; from music, literature, theatre, and even architectural plans. I was at home alone all day so I always had plenty of time and the work kept me active. My assignments came back with good marks, and I quickly signed up for a higher-level course focusing on the Renaissance the following year.

In 1998, I took a camera, notepad and pen and began researching the names on the village war memorial. *Among the First* is the forgotten story of the village's war memorial, the vicar that commissioned it, the mason who made it, the names commemorated upon it, and one that wasn't. Using army war diaries, church records, newspaper articles and even a ship's log, I was able to follow each man through his last moments. My painstaking and comprehensive research uncovered lost photographs and revealed much new information. In 2014, to mark the hundredth anniversary of the start of the Great War, I updated and donated my work to the villagers of Barford St Michael and submitted a copy to the Oxfordshire archive, and the Soldiers of Oxfordshire Museum in Woodstock in 2018.

Helen had applied to Oxford, Durham, and York and had done very well in her A-levels. She was awarded a prestigious scholarship to read philosophy, politics and economics at New College, Oxford, and was to start that September. A lucky break for me as Durham and York were far from home for both of us. Although Oxford was 20 miles away, my dad worked there so I was able to get lifts with him. Even though we were on different trajectories, I wanted to keep up with Helen for as long as I could. We agreed to make a long-distance relationship work. I feared that different lifestyles and Helen's expanding new world would bring a natural end to our three-year relationship.

During her studies, we had agreed that we limited our contact to weekends, holidays, and phone calls. Anthony moved out to live with his girlfriend, so his large bedroom was converted into a games room. I had plenty to keep me busy during the day; a PlayStation was installed and some of the village lads would come around to spend the evenings playing *Wipeout, FIFA 96*, and smoke pot with me. Still playing *Dungeons & Dragons*, my friend Gary would come and pick me up, help me to his car and take me the few miles to where we played and bring me home again, often staying for a few hours to chat. My dad had developed his interest in home cinema. Using powerful speakers, the crockery in the kitchen cupboards rattled with the explosions of the action films he watched vicariously. For him, a film had to have a car chase and an exploding helicopter to be any good.

How I first met my trusty sidekick! (A wheelchair)

I grew up in the '80s, unaware of disability. In my family, my cousin was born with a harelip and cleft palate which was resolved by surgery in childhood. My grandma faced down various physical problems with great stoicism as she reached the end of her life. These are two valid approaches to disability: pay for surgery to mitigate it, or bear it with dignity, but in both, disability is seen as a surmountable problem. This attitude ran through society too. *Children in Need* began portraying disabled people as tragic victims needing the kindness of others to survive 1980 and every year since. Joey Deacon, an elderly disabled man with cerebral palsy, appeared on *Blue Peter* in 1981. Although he was there to raise the profile of disability, his appearance only served to cruelly ridicule disabled people in playgrounds across the country.

Although it never occurred to me until much later, my Catholic upbringing had perpetuated the idea that disability was an affliction, a punishment for sin and could be visited on someone or cured by the power of God Himself. The message for me (and most of us who grew up in '80s Britain) was that *other people* agreed that disability is a terrible burden that only medical experts, a miracle, or money can relieve. For me, the wheelchair was the symbol of dependency, a pathetic surrender at the end of life. It stood squarely in the way of the 'normal' life I wanted. I didn't know anyone who used a wheelchair. I had always struggled with the shame I would feel at this act of surrender.

My mobility was worsening, and Helen saw me using a wheelchair as a practical solution. A small breakthrough came in summer 1998, on a holiday with her family. Although I could still 'walk' 100m from a parked car with assistance, I arranged to hire a wheelchair in Bordeaux, so I had a little more capacity in the hot weather on days out. I went along with this because I would be in a safe environment, where nobody knew me. I used this awkward contraption begrudgingly and as little as possible.

With grief, you have to hit the lowest point before you can pick yourself up and start to come back. You are truly blessed if someone loves you enough to hold your hand as you fall. My lowest point came when my mobility had deteriorated to the point where my quality of life had become much worse than what I thought would happen to me if I 'accepted' using a wheelchair. It was a very hard, very important lesson for me to learn. It is one that I have seen other people struggling with in their own life-changing moments. Helen caught me and still holds my hand, which I am incredibly grateful for.

Helen was having trouble fitting in at Oxford. Perhaps that strengthened our relationship at a time when Helen needed to feel reassured. I knew from my cousins that living and working with people from a public school background could be difficult. She would be an outsider herself. For example, early in her degree, Helen was advised by one of her tutors to write 'in a more thrusting style.' Our bond grew as I visited weekly and she would come home at weekends. In Oxford, Helen would meet me at the main entrance of her college and help me walk to her flat. In her second year, her room was off the main courtyard. There was a door on the outer wall that would have reduced the distance I had to walk. When Helen enquired about getting a key, she was told it was a fellow's door and that only fellows of the college were allowed to use it. I was surprised when I was dropped off outside the college a few weeks later and the door was propped open. As I watched, a wheelbarrow pushed by a builder emerged. I assumed he wasn't a fellow of the college. It was my first taste of ableism, and it summed up Oxford University's duty of care to its students. Fortunately, there were outsiders like Helen who had also made it there. Lovely, intelligent and gifted people like Helen. They became friends, but I felt they all barely survived at Oxford rather than flourished. This anger at the way Helen and her friends had been treated by their university convinced me that better student representation was required.

When Helen came back one weekend, we went to a supermarket on the edge of town. Pretending to be grown-ups, we picked up supplies for the weekend as usual. I was busy with my Open University studies and research and writing. I'd pretty much not been anywhere except the village pub. We pulled up in the supermarket car park one weekend. 'Why don't you try one of those chairs?' she asked brightly in her ever-practical way. I felt the usual angry response rising, yet this time it was different. I had had enough of being left behind and knew that I was in danger of being left alone forever. Encouraged by the very small possibility of seeing anybody I knew, this time I agreed to try. Helen duly wheeled one of the basic contrivances over, with squeaking castors and its footplates clumsily adjusted to different heights. I insisted she walk next to me and not push; in case it gave the wrong impression to all the people I thought would be watching.

Slowly and anxiously, I wheeled myself through the car park. Once we entered the supermarket, everything changed. I was overwhelmed by my new freedom. Whizzing down the aisles, popping items into the basket on my lap, weighing up the offers; making my own choices again. I couldn't believe how silly I'd been. I had let my deep shame of being disabled stop me living and trap me inside my home like an angry spider. My life changed forever that day. Today, I realise with a wry smile that that Richard was blissfully unaware that he still couldn't reach most of the products, that the accessible toilet probably doubled as a storeroom, and that the staff probably wouldn't have been trained to offer him any assistance!

My Open University foundation course had a residential element. A week of living on campus and going to lectures. I was prepared to use a wheelchair throughout, mainly because it was held at Reading University, where nobody would know me. Home for the summer, Helen came along as my personal assistant. Five days of using a wheelchair, living as a full-time student, and going to classes (and the bar!) confirmed for me that I would thrive at university.

During the holidays, we visited Paris, Berlin, and San Sebastian with Helen's parents and did our own travelling – exciting weekend breaks in European cities. I took the wheelchair and was glad of the anonymity. I was slowly becoming more comfortable but also more dependent on it. We visited Amsterdam, Rome, Dublin, Prague, and Vienna. Something of a grand tour. Our trip to Rome was especially memorable. Arriving in Rome at night, we decided to walk to our hotel near the Vatican. At the end of a street was the Colosseum, lit up as you've seen it in a thousand movies. Tired from the flight and the unexpected late-night walk across hilly Rome, Helen argued that we should press on, as what we were looking at was just a fake Colosseum. It wasn't. When we did go to the 'real' Colosseum, we found it had a glass lift installed. It became my go-to example for many years of how effective access can be integrated seamlessly into ancient buildings. Especially helpful when discussing access with owners of listed buildings. But the more I thought about it, the more I realised that the lift was not installed during the twilight years of John Paul II's papacy because of general altruism – but thanks to the money and influence of one disabled person.

We went to the Vatican on our last day, to see its many exquisite works of art and the Sistine Chapel. At the very top of the museum was the beginning of a huge spiral ramp. I was so excited – it was an opportunity I could not miss. Helen pointed to a sign at the top of the ramp showing a wheelchair user with a red cross over it. A clear instruction forbidding wheelchair users to use the ramp. 'That's just for old people who can't handle their speed!' I replied dismissively and began my descent. Going down the first few floors was fine but I couldn't see very far ahead because of the crowd. I was surprised by a jolt, then another a few metres later. They were getting deeper and closer together and turning into – steps! Too late to turn back, I stopped, embarrassed and terrified. 'Can we help?' asked a voice with a thick Northern Irish accent from behind me. I turned. The 'we' was a gang of middle-aged nuns. The correct term is a 'superfluity', but I prefer 'gang' – it makes them sound dangerous!

Remembering how tough nuns were from my time at primary school, I thanked them. With Helen, they picked up my chair and carried me down the rest of the stairs. As I looked at their stoic, slowly reddening faces, I felt like I was the Pope being borne aloft by grunting angels. Maybe they felt I was their penance. I later learned that this was the Bramante Staircase, designed by Giuseppe Momo in 1932.

Back in the square, guards admitted the multitudes with tickets into St Peter's Basilica. Deciding to push our luck, we joined the queue and, before reaching the front, we were waved through some corridors to a lift. The stewards were obviously used to working with wheelchair users. I had been in several cathedrals and many churches, but this was the biggest church in the world. Michelangelo himself had worked many years on the building and died before it was finished. This place had inspired the spread of the Catholic religion all over the world. I felt deep connection. We ended up in a side chapel with a lot of people, mostly nuns. Soon, an announcement was made that, due to rain, the Pope would now be giving his audience from where we were. It was like having a backstage pass at a pop concert; we were swept along by an ensuing rush of nuns to some barriers at one end of the room. An excited hush fell ... a door opened and the Pope came out in his electric throne. I couldn't help it; he reminded me of Davros, Emperor of the Daleks. He looked so withered and tired. He stopped, hand raised weakly in a blessing in our general direction. I felt that he was absolving me personally, that the Catholic church and I were finally even. More importantly, I had learned that even if you don't have the right ticket, a bit of entitlement and confidence (and a wheelchair) can get you where you need to be.

Next stop: Amsterdam! We were so taken by Amsterdam that we returned a couple of times. Obviously, the cannabis culture and the flat landscape appealed, but it was the social freedom and the lack of shame that struck me. On a busy shopping street, you would have a greengrocer next to a sex shop. I loved watching old ladies carefully examine the local garden produce, then peruse the display of dildos in the shop window next door with equal interest.

One New Year's Eve, we quickly found the city centre bars were ticket-only or completely full. Eventually, we saw a couple leave one bar, so we went in, assuming we could take their seats. We brought drinks from a friendly barman and sat down. I glanced around, wondering why Helen was the only woman in the bar. I quickly realised: the racks of tourist information were all gay-themed. We were in a gay bar! Deciding that there were other people who were more deserving of our seats, we finished our drinks and left to see in the New Year from our hotel room at The Cok City Hotel. Hurrying across Dam Square, we became aware of the Dutch tradition of throwing firecrackers on the ground around people's feet. I found this stressful enough, without my wheels getting stuck in the tramlines.

We explored these cities by foot and only occasionally using public transport, since I was physically still able to transfer myself well. We sometimes used taxis. The best taxis were in Prague. Where we found, for example, a lovely old Soviet-era Trabant (they were everywhere!), whose shabby interior was decorated with pornographic playing cards and with what we assumed were several neat bullet holes in the windscreen. After pulling over and explaining our hotel was on a one-way street, our swarthy driver grinned, looked over his shoulder and hurtled down it in reverse.

I began to realise that a wheelchair is a tool to explore the world and does not define the person using it. Combined with the confidence I developed thanks to Helen and her family, I was ready for the next step.

OFF HE GOES

By the end of 1999, I had passed three courses and earned a diploma with the Open University. I was desperate to catch up with my peers, who had started university four years before. I knew this qualification would not be enough for me to join Helen at Oxford, but I hoped it would appeal to a more modern institution. Helen's aunt suggested I try Oxford Brookes University. Far from me having to convince them that I was good enough, the university staff assured me that I would be very welcome there, promised I would have everything I needed, and encouraged me to apply. I started in the second year of a BA in Modern History in September 2000. At 24, I was older than most students and, thanks to my experience with the Open University, I knew I had picked a course I would love. I applied for a place in halls too, knowing from my recent summer school stay at Reading University, that I would be able to enjoy the social experience and make the move from home. I excitedly started to work through my reading list over the summer.

I was first to arrive at my new flat and waited nervously to greet my new flatmates with a cup of tea. Would I be able to fit it in? Would they see the wheelchair instead of me? I needn't have worried. First was Dave, a man's man with a heart of gold. Next was Tom, a charming, well-spoken guy, then Melanie from Bordeaux, and Asami from Japan. Thanks to all of them, our flat was always full of people. The very first night, there was a fire alarm and all of us were milling around in the chilly night air. Some of the male students were wearing brightly coloured, badly fitting dressing gowns – obviously borrowed in haste from the female students they were spending the night with. What a great way to meet people!

My course was modular so it was possible to study quite a broad range of areas. The modules on offer for my course were entirely based in/on subjects that had had a significant effect on the twentieth century. At the end of each module was an exam or an essay. I studied Irish history, feminist history and local history, but my favourites were the modules on fascism and 20th-century German history. I had really enjoyed Professor Roger Griffin's books on fascism and was fascinated by the way he taught with such passion and energy. His lectures were like stand-up routines, full of personal stories, observations, and call backs. Quite taken with him, I would talk about him all the time and encouraged Helen to come to one of his lectures.

Almost the opposite was the very austere Professor of German history, Dr Detlef Muhlberger. Also renowned in his field, his command of sources to support his arguments was breathtaking. The History Department at Brookes had a better government rating than its counterpart at Oxford. I developed an interest in eugenics, especially medical killing in Nazi Germany. For instance, how 250,000 disabled people were murdered. The gas vans used to kill many of them were the precursor to the gas chambers of the Holocaust.

Right from the first day, I wanted to support and represent my fellow disabled students. At the end of the first term, I was elected as a disabled students' representative. This involved contributing to a termly forum. I spent my time with Tom, my flatmate, or working. At the weekends, Helen or friends from home would visit. We'd spend many evenings and mornings at Morals, the Students' Union's bar. Sometimes going there for breakfast in the mornings, and not leaving until the end of that night. I managed to cook basic meals, but drank and smoked more in that year than I had ever before or since.

In the name of health and safety, I was required to position myself at the front of my lectures near the entrance. As a result, I would often find they were being delivered directly to me. This was usually fine; I was there to learn and grateful for that. Still, sometimes, on warm afternoons, I could feel my eyes start to close. I would sometimes have to bite my tongue to keep myself awake. Nothing to do with my late nights, of course.

Returning home for Christmas, my parents informed me that they were moving to the Isle of Wight. They were downsizing to live by the coast and my brother and I would be welcome to come for holidays. The news was a bit of a shock. Pat was still living at home, so he would have to go with them. This was the start of a series of ill-fated moves that saw them move back to Oxfordshire, down to Devon, and then over to Ireland. It felt to me like they were chasing the fantasy of a happy seaside retirement. They deserved some happiness, but their problems would follow them and eventually the process of moving would begin again.

Helen had taken a summer job allocating accommodation at the university. As I was staying in halls, she made sure I had a series of 'interesting' flatmates to keep me company. One was Andris from Latvia. I remember, and this isn't a joke, that he was moved to tears when he saw the fresh fruit on display at the supermarket we took him to. I helped him write a CV that lauded him as one of the foremost experts in carpet fitting in Latvia!

The social model of disability

At the end of my first year, I was elected as the students with disabilities officer for my final year. With my coursework, a dissertation, and an exchange overseas coming up, I didn't really have much time to devote to it, nonetheless it set me on the path to becoming a full-time student officer after I graduated. Wrongly believing that disabled people should give their time and expertise for free, I do remember unsuccessfully trying to convince Dame Tanni Grey Thompson, former wheelchair racer, to come and give a motivational talk and being quite upset when I didn't hear back from her. However, some interesting training I attended as part of this role changed my life.

I was used to observing social phenomena from different philosophical viewpoints, in spite of that I had never heard of the 'social model of disability.' It was an epiphany. It drew a clear distinction between impairment and disability. According to it, disability does not belong to any one of us but consists of the barriers that a person with an impairment experiences as a result of the way in which society – with its perceptions of shame, sickness and helplessness – is organised that excludes or devalues them. That I cannot access a service or use a feature doesn't disable me; it is society's failure to provide universal access and its acceptance that I cannot participate in society that does.

It is a surprisingly recent idea. In 1976 in the UK, The Union of Physically Impaired Against Segregation (UPIAS) published its Fundamental Principles of Disability. These became its manifesto and a seminal document for the British disabled people's movement. Pioneer Mike Oliver developed these ideas in the 1983 book Social Work with Disabled People. He used Marxism to frame the story of disabled people in Britain. During the 18th century, industrialisation exposed disabled people to the forces of capitalism and dictated such individuals to be unproductive, which led to them being forced outside of the family into institutions. This has led to 250 years of stigma and oppression as disabled people continue to be excluded from society. This limited focus on the economic value of disabled people can be seen in the policies of successive governments.

This blew my mind and changed the way I see myself and others. Seeing disability in this way sets you free; it lifts the burden of guilt from the disabled person, but it also exposes you to all the ableism and ignorance behind it. The impairment may be yours, but my educational experience taught me that disability is other people.

STUDY ABROAD

Cinder block walls, metal beds, hard floor,
bought a lamp, a phone, chalk for our door,
drew thin curtains and pushed beds together,
made a little home, a true endeavour.
With no distractions I listened and read,
joining the program, looking straight ahead.
Was learning so much and lifting the veil,
The day that spartan womb became our jail
when I believed the whole world went insane,
that we were never going home again.
I met brave New York, shivering and cowed,
Mourning her fallen, then, suddenly proud,
an easy reckoning, someone to blame.
I got home, but we were never the same.

'Rhode Island Sonnet' – Richard Brown

Study Abroad

In my final year, I applied to do an exchange in America. After considering universities in Colorado (too cold) and California (too big), I chose the University of Rhode Island (URI). If you're wondering, the tiny state of Rhode Island is on the North-East coast of America, part of New England. A former state college, URI was a similar size to Brookes and not pretentious like its posh Ivy League neighbour, Brown University. (I did visit my namesake, Brown University, if only to gaze through its ornate gates.) URI was just like Brookes, and I had a good feeling about the place. I was excited about visiting nearby New York and Boston and witnessing the kaleidoscope beauty of the gold and reds of fall there. Helen had just graduated with a 2:1, which she says was one of the greatest disappointments of her life. I thought it was a very respectable result, as a bright comprehensive school student in such an archaic environment, but she felt she had let herself down and clearly needed a rest. As our experiences travelling together made me feel confident that Helen and I could live for four months in America together, I arranged a direct payment to cover the costs of her coming along as my helper/note taker. URI was a 'dry' campus, in terms of alcohol not the weather, and as it was quite remote, I found plenty of time to read all my course books and re-read the notes Helen had taken in my classes. Embarrassingly, my grades were the best I had ever known. I was fascinated to see how Black Power politics, the Holocaust, Soviet History and cultural anthropology were taught in America.

We stayed in an all-female dorm, with our own en-suite toilet and shower, soon making friends with our neighbours. We had to travel everywhere by bus, but on a shopping trip to the state capital, Providence, and being over the age of 21, we managed to pick up a six-pack of beer and hide it in our wardrobe. Some of the lectures were early, so our routine was to cross the quad before breakfast, after drinking vending-machine Dr Pepper instead of coffee. We signed up for all the exchange student activities, such as a trip to a Red Sox game in Boston and a spooky Halloween experience in a warehouse with live actors to add an extra level of scariness. As we trundled around, a witch broke character and leaned down to whisper: 'Mind out, dear, there are some steps over there.' Outside, my chair broke. I made it back to the minibus and spent the rest of the evening being told by our driver about how limousines are made. Helen bravely continued the evening without me, and got to meet world champion wrestler Trish Stratus.

We also took full part in college life: made weird friends, went to college football games and pep rallies, joined the college improv society, and went along to a talk given by local spiritualists. A film distributor piloted a horror movie called *Th13teen Ghosts* in one of the lecture theatres to gauge student reaction. Like many things, watching films in America is a different prospect to doing the same thing in Britain. American audiences, especially young people, are much more invested, with clapping, cheering and interacting. The film went down well and was distributed successfully across the world. We also knew that this wasn't just a college or horror genre thing as when we saw *Lord of the Rings* in a mainstream cinema, there were people in the queue dressed up as characters from the film and shouting and clapping at all the big moments.

There were two professors who I am particularly grateful to have learned so much from. Professor Robert G. Weisbord was my teacher for Holocaust studies. A 67-year-old Jewish New Yorker, a snappy dresser, and an excellent storyteller. He was a civil rights pioneer himself, being the first to teach a class on African-American studies in a New England University in 1967. His class sought to refocus Nazi oppression as open racism and sought to understand how ordinary people enabled this regime. When calling the register, he referred to the other students by their surname but always called me 'Richard' as a sign of respect. An accomplished storyteller, he would often colour his stories with personal anecdotes and add obscure Yiddish words. In keeping with his post-modernist approach, he would end his thorough lectures with a big sigh and say, 'Well, we just don't know.'

To this day, I think of him and smile. Like all good teachers, he left a profound mark on me. There was one story in particular that comes to mind. He had a friend who was so risk-averse he wore a helmet on his exercise bike. This friend would bitterly complain that he never won anything on the lottery, but never bought a ticket. I can still hear Professor Weisbord whisper, 'You gotta buy a ticket, Richard, you gotta buy a ticket.' The messages I took from this were: some people just like to feel sorry for themselves and you have to make good things happen. This is wisdom to live by.

The second teacher I am particularly grateful for is Professor Peniel Joseph who taught the class on Black Power. Today, he is a professor at the LBJ School of Public Affairs and the History Department in the College of Liberal Arts at the University of Texas, Austin. He is also the founding director of the school's Centre for the Study of Race and Democracy. He encouraged my understanding of the similarities between race and disability and their links to poverty and struggle for equality. I had studied the relationship between empire and slavery in Britain, yet never comprehended the struggle for Black dignity that had been raging in America for the last 400 years. Knowing little about Black American History, I read hungrily about amazing people I'd never encountered before: Stokely Carmichael, Robert F. Williams, Huey Newton, Bobby Seale, Harriet Tubman, and Fred Hampton.

I studied the Black Panther Party in some depth. Although notorious for their militancy, the Panthers also established food kitchens, schools, medical centres, and a newspaper to empower Black people all over America. The Panthers were influenced by Maoism and were encouraged to read and follow Mao's *Little Red Book* (Tse-Tung, 2018) to set up 'survival programmes' within their communities and take their message around the world. This was the first time I had thought about the 'intersectionality' between all groups engaged in the global struggle against poverty. Just a few months before, I had learnt about the social model of disability and our own struggle for equality.

Intersectionality

While studying, I read an article called 'Black Like Mao', exploring the links between Maoism and Black Power. Essentially, Marxist thinking promised justice for those oppressed by capitalism through revolution. It appealed to many revolutionary groups in the '60s and '70s. In 1967, Robert Williams, a key figure in the civil rights movement, announced: 'Chairman Mao is the first world leader to elevate our people's struggle to the fold of the world revolution.' Mao was calling for a global revolution against the forces of capitalism and hoped that a large group of oppressed Americans would join him. Mao was not saying that he was Black, but that he understood and knew what it was to struggle against oppression. I also learned how the international debates of Martin Luther King Jr. and Malcolm X enabled audiences to see global connections between the struggles of Black people against poverty in America and against colonial powers around the world.

I began to understand that although discrimination is felt differently by every individual, we can share how that feels. We can use that shared experience to stand together against it. Several years later, I recalled this universalisation of discrimination when I contributed, on behalf of Birmingham City Council, to the White Paper which led to The Equalities Act (2010). It bought together 116 different pieces of legislation and created nine protected groups: Age, Disability, Gender Reassignment, Marriage and Civil Partnership, Pregnancy and Maternity, Race, Religion or Belief, Sex, and Sexual Orientation. Discrimination against any of these groups was unlawful, but the act recognised discrimination itself as a single act, with many different types possible.

Being a straight White male with an obvious disability is my unique intersectional identity and determines my experiences of disadvantage and privilege. Twitter (rebranded 'X' in 2023), has enabled me to hear the voices and stories of members of other groups. I soon realised that although I could not know how discrimination feels for every individual, I could use my experiences to empathise with them. I have always felt a strong link with any other oppressed group and am painfully aware of their struggle.

A film I saw recently highlighted the deep links between Black and disabled lives. Produced by the Obamas, *Crip Camp: A Disability Revolution* (Newnham, 2020) tells the story of a group of young adults who are thrown together at a summer camp for the handicapped in America in 1971. Many have to be carried from the inaccessible coaches they arrive on. Then, in the first truly inclusive environment of their lives, they undergo an awakening and discover that their disabilities are created by other people and enforced through the environment around them. Early in the film, a Black counsellor talks about how he knew from a young age to never look a White policeman in the eye. He talks about how struck he is by the similarity of how his disabled companions were also made to feel inferior to others. This gives a hint that there is common ground between the prejudices faced by Black and disabled people. A point that is made very clearly later in the same documentary.

In April 1977, disabled protesters were occupying a government building in San Francisco. With this revelation and inspired by the civil rights movement, this group of friends formed a diverse and fully inclusive organisation and began a fifteen-year fight for equality for all disabled people. They protested, resisted, and occupied; they fearlessly put themselves in harm's way and drew support from other marginalised groups at the same time. Amongst them was Bradley Lomax, a member of the Black Panther Party with multiple sclerosis. As the occupation stretched into its eleventh day, the protesters, with their own ingenuity and support from other groups, were kept going with hot meals supplied by none other than the Black Panther Party from their kitchen in nearby Oakland. When asked why they were giving their support, they explained, 'We're all trying to make the world a better place; if you care enough to sleep on the floor here, then we're going to help you.' The FBI tried to stop these deliveries; the Black Panthers held their ground. The daily deliveries continued until the protest ended successfully on the 25th day.

One of the proudest moments of my life came when Professor Joseph handed back an essay I had written, looked me in the eye and said, 'Richard, you're with the program.' Brimming with confidence for the first time in my life, I wrote a prize-winning essay about the strengths of equality and diversity and gave a stirring speech to the URI Students' Union about living with disability. This confidence is what I have taken with me into any discussion about equality ever since.

There's going to be a war!

But the most profound lesson came just days after we arrived. On a Tuesday morning in 2001, some 176 miles from us, two airliners hit the World Trade Centre towers in New York. As we left the dining hall after breakfast through the unusually silent kitchen, the staff had gathered around a small TV. 'There's going to be a war,' predicted one as we passed. Sensing the atmosphere, we didn't interrupt to ask why. As we watched the TV coverage in our common room throughout that morning, the footage repeated, and then mixed with new material, so it became difficult to follow exactly what had happened or if this was only the beginning. Our friends left to go home and be with their loved ones. Understandably, everything seemed to change overnight and US flags appeared everywhere. Suddenly, I felt very aware that I wasn't an American. We were advised to stay on campus while the FBI examined the records of foreign students studying politics. I assumed this included mine. As all planes were grounded and war loomed, it was the furthest from home I'd ever felt. On the day after the attacks, we went to a hastily organised Stop The War demo on campus – we were the only people who turned up. It was obviously just too soon.

I was so glad that Helen was there with me. Her misjudgement of the situation did lead to a few problems! Like all the other rooms in our dorm, there was a chalkboard on our door so that we could let our neighbours know where we were. Soon after the attacks, Helen went to pick up pizza on the campus, leaving me studying in the room. Unbeknownst to me, she had drawn a grinning cartoon bun full of currents, wearing Saudi headdress, and labelled it 'Bun Laden.' I could hear an angry crowd growing outside the door, both male and female voices chattering. I heard phrases like 'That's fucked up, man' and occasional sharp thumps on the door. Sensing the growing tension, I wondered what was going on and if I was about to get lynched. Luckily, one of the seniors living in the dorm calmed the situation down, explaining that we were lovely British people, who had made a clumsy, misguided attempt at humour and did not mean to offend. The crowd dispersed peacefully before Helen cheerfully returned with our dinner.

In the days after the attacks, Helen regularly phoned her parents. She agreed with them that America had brought the attacks on itself through years of failed foreign policy. From the course on Black politics, we knew similar opinions had been expressed during the Vietnam War. While I totally agreed with her, I wondered if it was the best thing to say over the phone while extra attention was being paid to us as foreign students. New York was still in shock and we had planned to spend a day there a few days after the attacks. We still went, unsure if we were going as mourners or tourists as we drifted our way down Manhattan Island. It was like a tomb, preternaturally quiet, with the ground covered in dark acrid dust, which soon covered my wheels and hands. As we neared Ground Zero, the smoke became unbearable and we were given face masks to wear. We often passed firehouses with boards outside displaying photographs of the brave men and women who had not made it back.

In this time of loss, my grandma died. I missed her funeral, so was glad that we had been to visit her in hospital before we left. I felt the long, rambling, and heartfelt conversation we had then was an satisfactory goodbye. Thankfully, our parents came to visit us as planned, braving a transatlantic flight just weeks later. Helen's dad, John, hired and drove a minivan across New England, stopping in Boston where my 'metric' wheelchair broke dramatically and had to be repaired by my dad with hastily purchased 'imperial' parts and tools. Back in New York, we tried again to be tourists. With my mum keen to see places that were important to John Lennon, we visited the Strawberry Fields memorial in Central Park and the Dakota building. As a dark, autumn chill crept over Central Park, I felt Lennon's presence as I imagined his last moments. We also went to the Guggenheim Museum and even went to a Broadway show.

Although this was our second visit to New York, stark reminders of the attacks were everywhere. When we looked down on the city lights from atop the Empire State Building, the wreckage of Ground Zero still smouldered. On a cruise around the harbour, the chill sea air still carried the sickly smell of burning that we recognised from our previous trip. Our hotel (like every other in New York) was full of firefighters from all over America. Our elevator to breakfast stopped at each floor, gradually filling up with firefighters, solemnly silent in their dress uniforms, on their way to a memorial service to say goodbye to their fallen colleagues.

The attacks had shown me that life is very precious. Helen and I had been together five years and she was the one I wanted to be with forever. She finally acquiesced to my frequent pressing for us to get married. I had already made the emotional commitment, but for Helen, it was a massive life decision which deserved proper consideration. Now she told me she had made her decision. On a weekend trip to Canada, we picked an antique platinum and diamond eternity ring and I tried to find somewhere appropriate for such an important moment. We found a salubrious-looking Chinese restaurant and asked for a table for two. Instead, we were hastily shown to a noisy buffet room with metal benches. It was full of multi-generational Chinese families having lunch. There were no waiters or menus, just a jug of tap water on each table. It didn't occur to me to question this as I was so focused on going through with the proposal. How to phrase it? I had no plan and absolutely nothing to offer apart from love. I knew that, thanks to her, I had embarked on an amazing journey. I didn't know where it would take me, but I wanted her to be my partner on it and for us to bring children into the world together. Just like in this restaurant, Helen must have known that she wouldn't be getting the best table in a life with me, but our lives together would never be ordinary either. Getting down on one knee might have been out of the question, but she said yes. She hadn't changed her mind!

We enjoyed a final visit to New York, taking the subway past the Brooklyn Bridge to Coney Island; spending the unusually sunny winter afternoon walking along the boardwalk and visiting the aquarium. The run-down funfair felt so familiar, just as we had seen in so many films. We felt that New York had finally welcomed us. Just before we were due to return to the UK, we hired a car to do some last-minute sightseeing and to say goodbye to some friends from our dorm who had already gone home for the holidays. Plans changed because disaster struck! On our road trip, we had a low-speed collision with traffic waiting to turn right. In the confused moments after the accident, I could not see well (my glasses had flown off) except for smoke billowing through the central console. Somebody was tapping at the window, asking if we were OK.

I was absolutely furious. I didn't realise that we had *caused* the accident. The police arrived and checked us for injuries. Still very much in shock, Helen rode in the front of the squad car with the officer, while I rolled around on the hard-plastic back seat. At the station, one of the officers called the hire company to tell them the car we had been driving had been written off. He hung up and shook his head. 'It was only two weeks old,' we heard him tell a colleague. Because we had followed Helen's dad's sage advice and paid extra for full insurance, the whole incident only cost us about £50 and a few scratches. Understandably, the hire company weren't able to give us a new car, so we took a taxi back to the state capital, Providence, and booked into a hotel until our flights home in a few days.

Back in Oxford, I worked hard for the rest of my final year. I began my dissertation on Nazi family policy and the state-sponsored murder of disabled Germans, and how this foreshadowed the Holocaust and that the allies knew it was happening. I had to translate many of the articles I needed from their original German. One of my random flatmates the previous summer had been German and he connected me with German-speaking friends of his in Oxford. The winter mornings were dark when I woke and went to the library and dark again when I got back to my room. If not for weekends, I could have been a vampire!

Realising how valuable my experience was and with a new chapter of my life beginning, I wanted to encourage others to experience what I had. I stood for election in the Students' Union Executive Committee as the deputy president with a responsibility for welfare. It was a one-year sabbatical (salaried) post. My campaign slogan was 'Get Rich Quick!' and my publicity photo was me sitting in my wheelchair with a coin superimposed where the wheel should have been. I did a little campaigning, promising better representation, especially for students living in university accommodation, and continuing to oppose tuition fees. I was elected unopposed to serve for the year following my graduation. My first proper job.

During my last term, I applied to the homeless register. I explained that after the last day of my halls contract, we would have nowhere to live. I explained my needs and that my parents had moved away. Towards the end of my accommodation contract, we viewed a spacious flat in a new development just off Oxford's famously cosmopolitan Cowley Road that we had been offered as temporary accommodation. It was a brand-new flat; the paint was still drying! Amazingly, we would only pay a rent relative to our earnings. We would be the first people in the building and could move in on return from our honeymoon. I was confident we would be there for a long time, as accessible ground-floor properties were rarely available.

I was incredibly proud when I graduated from university. Oxford Brookes had supported me and my time there changed my life and shaped my future. Most importantly, I felt valued as a person. This was distinctly opposite to the truly medieval attitudes to disability I had experienced down the hill at Oxford University, and shows what a difference the attitudes of our institutions can make.

The media, freedom of speech, and false equivalence

The mainstream media is responsible for the othering of groups, spreading fear and misinformation and misreporting the world around us. So, when Oxford

Brookes asked me to feature in a piece for the local media, I knew instinctively what the right story was. I was simply a student who had accomplished a difficult challenge through his own hard work and with the proper support. So, I wrote a carefully worded account carefully explaining how the university had supported me. I met the photographer on graduation day to have my picture taken. When the finished articles were published, guess what? Both followed the personal-tragedy model of disability, or, as it is often known, full-on inspo-porn – when a disabled person is considered an inspiration for doing something quite ordinary. 'Overcoming the Odds for Cap and Gown' and 'Degree of Willpower' stated the headlines. I was disappointed, but didn't complain because at least it was some recognition. I just shrugged my shoulders and carried on. I realise now that this article strengthened the othering of disabled people and the already low expectations that 'ableds' have for us. I was part of the problem.

A heady nationalist myth of British resilience and nostalgia has long been played on by our politicians and media. We like to look back on the fantasy of a golden age as a simpler, better time. The Blitz is held as a defining moment when people worked together, as it slips from public memory that crime went up by 57% during it. British people have been fed compelling myths from the exploits of Francis Drake (English, 2023), Winston Churchill (English, 2022) and the character of James Bond (Higgs,

2022) that reinforce the stereotype of the resolute and plucky Brit at the centre of events. Experts are ignored; displaying empathy is dismissed as empty 'virtue signalling'; and a nanny state/immigrants/Europe are taking away our freedom/jobs/fish. A lot of fear and unseen 'woke' enemies are used to divide people, create fear and, worse, apathy. It is such apathy that makes us look inwards and remain locked in a system that fails to treat all of its citizens as equals.

Disabled people are especially let down badly. The media perpetuates the myths that disabled people are an unproductive, burdensome minority. A survey into the press's portrayal of disability in a ground-breaking survey in 2012 found that three-quarters of disabled people believed the volume of negativity was 'significantly increasing', with 9 out of 10 saying that there was a link between the negative press portrayal of disabled people and rising hostility and hate crime. Things have not got better since. In 2021, the Disability Unit's UK Disability Survey research report found that 54% of disabled people were worried about being insulted or harassed in the street or any other public place. This is due in part to the sensationalism of the media, and also the ableism and ignorance of those in positions of power.

Disabled people are not the only victims; there is something more malevolent going on. Consider the appalling treatment meted out by the media that saw Amanda Knox wrongly convicted for murder. As Frances Ryan concluded in a March 2019 piece on disability hate crime in *The Guardian*: 'Huge swathes of the media have normalised hatred and suspicion of minorities for years.' I agree. As human beings, we are responsible for recognising and rejecting these tired tropes. We must demand better. Equally, journalists who are in the privileged position of portraying any minority group have a much greater responsibility to reject such lazy and damaging clichés. Media bias is rife with many large organisations reflecting the views of their right-wing owners.

Universities play an important part in developing a global view and exposing such threats. Students' Unions had a policy of not giving a platform to openly racist or fascist groups. Speakers such as Nigel Farage, Nick Griffin and George Galloway were rightly denied an opportunity to speak at universities. Worryingly, the UK Government announced in February 2021 that universities have a duty to protect freedom of speech and have threatened to sanction those who don't. At first glance, this doesn't look like a problem, but it easily becomes one when 'freedom of speech' is confused with false equivalency, giving extreme opinions an equal standing with carefully researched views, as it has been in the mainstream media. Normalising right-wing rhetoric – giving it credibility – is dangerous.

Balance is important. A key part of the progress made by the civil rights movement in the '60s was university debate. Martin Luther King Jr. believed in finding equality through integration. Malcolm X (Haley, 1987) rejected this and believed in separatism. Although the two men never met on the debating circuit, Malcolm debated the issue of Black citizenship in American colleges with moderates like Bayard Rustin. Rustin advocated the integration of Black people into American society. Balance was provided by Malcolm X who talked about Black pride and demanded a separate state for Black people as they returned to Africa. He advocated violence if it was in self-defence. He was accused of being a dangerous hate-preacher and his visits were blocked by a few university administrations. This sparked protests around academic liberty and freedom of speech. People asked: who is doing the inviting, who is doing the 'cancelling' and why? Universities quickly understood that they could hold a compelling debate on a hot topic if they provided knowledgeable and credible speakers.

Balance can only be stretched so far. The universities were not expected to shift the focus of the issue by providing a White supremacist for 'balance'. Universities and their students must decide who should be given a platform to speak. Not the government.

CONCLUSION: RISE

Through Helen and her parents, and especially their strong socialist beliefs and work ethic, I got back that self-belief I had had in childhood. They helped restore my ambitions and encouraged me to follow them. Helen was so good for me. There was something in her personality that brought out the best in mine. Over the next few years, we formed a strong bond through weekend breaks in European capitals and immersion in popular culture. For the first time, I believed that I could do the things I had always wanted.

Going to university was life-changing. Alongside a wider political awakening through my coursework, I began to develop a strong belief in representation alongside a greater understanding of disability rights. I enjoyed my new independence. Most importantly, I grew as a person.

CONCLUSION: RISE

Vital to my progress was campus culture. Oxford Brookes University had kept its promises: it provided me with taxis from my accommodation to the campus every morning, employed fellow students to push me back again, allowed me to record my lectures, allowed extra time and a computer to type on in my exams, and supported me to take part in a student exchange in America in my final year. They had been flexible with my accommodation, allowing me to live in my ground-floor flat over the summers, and even stored my things when I was in America.

Also central to my educational experience – as it intensified my sense of achievement – was my American exchange. I will feel connected to all of the people we met and all of the places we explored forever. Being in an unfamiliar environment with its rich cultural heritage, I began to see disability as part of a much wider struggle for equality, I felt the chilling fear of being an outsider, found new confidence in my beliefs and my writing, and learned to value the wisdom of elders. Professor Weisbord's story about hopes not materialising without action and visiting New York in the days following 9/11 influenced me more deeply than I could imagine. Helen and I were getting married; she was key to every part of my awakening, and has held my hand every step of the way since.

Now I was ready and in my prime; my best years and the world were before me and, once again, there for me to make my own. I was understanding my special abilities now and felt a powerful desire to empower and represent others. My experience at Oxford Brookes Students' Union and the influence of Helen's parents set the tone for a career in the public sector. I knew what I wanted, and there was so much I needed to do. I had to make everything really matter, all in a much shorter time frame than the average person might expect. I had had a massive setback, but was on my way again. Watch out, world!

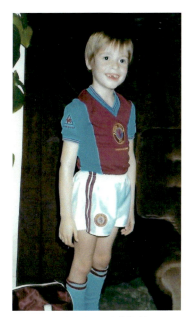

My 7th Birthday, Lichfield 1983

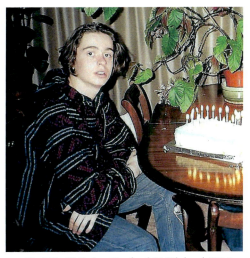

My 18th Birthday, Barford St Michael, 1994

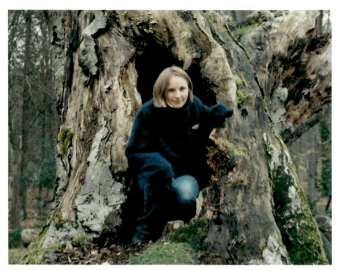

Somewhere in the New Forest 1996

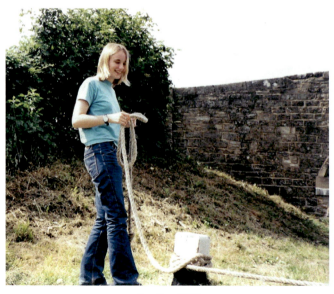

Boating 1997

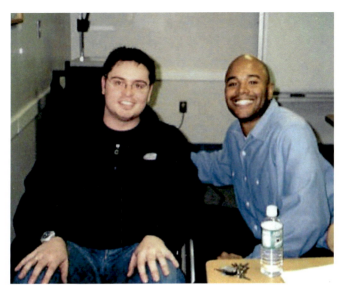

Professor Joseph and me, URI 2001

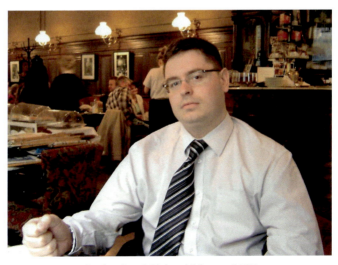

Professional Richard, Vienna, 2005

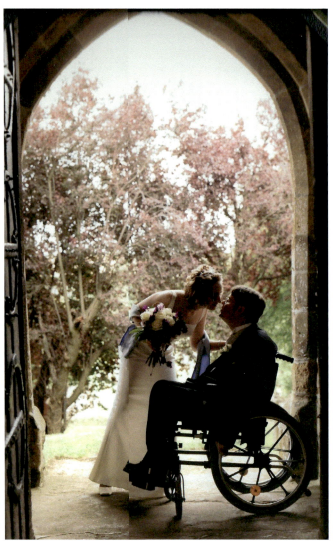

Married, Barford St Michael, 2002

Part Three

A Day In The Life

Over the next ten years, I continued to chase the things that I thought I wanted, but could never have. I had been to university and found a first home; there was still a family, a career, and driving to experience! They would complement each other and take us to new places!

ABSOLUTE BEGINNERS

The first thing to do was to start my own family. We booked a wedding date with the village church and I asked my dad to be my best man, so the task of organising my stag do fell to him. He asked me where I would like to go. I replied that as long as it was somewhere that was built recently and did not have loud music, I didn't mind. Taking this into account, he hired a minibus and drove us all out to Birmingham where we met up with my uncles, had dinner, and then went on to a gentlemen's club. My dad still maintains that he innocently thought a gentlemen's club was a place where everyone wore smoking jackets, smoked cigars, drank brandy, and read newspapers while sitting in high-backed armchairs – and was surprised to find it was not (pull the other one, Dad!). We were the first customers in there and pretty soon all of my friends were being propositioned by scantily clad ladies. My father-in-law, John, felt uncomfortable, excused himself, and went for a walk. I cannot say any more about that night as we were all sworn to secrecy on the way back. All I can say is everyone made it home, having spent all their money.

We were married in St Michael's church in Barford St Michael on a beautiful, warm, sunny day, the air full of blossom. With lots of help from Helen's dad, we worked hard to give our wedding a personal feel. We chose the hymns, including 'By Vows of Love Together Bound', a lovely North American hymn that I found on the internet. We printed our own invitations and orders of service, had a Shakespeare sonnet as a reading, and a solo violin performance from one of Helen's friends. The vicar was very good, having made a deep impression on me previously. Helen dropped the word 'obey' from her vows and decided to keep her own name, explaining that there was already a Helen Brown in our family. It took me a long time to fully understand her decision, feeling inadequate somehow. Now, I admire Helen for her 'Helen-ness'. It was her decision; I wasn't expected to change my name, so why should she?

The happiest day of my life did not start well. I'd asked to spend an extra few days in halls and everyone had gone home for the summer. My last night there was also the night before the wedding. In the morning, I could not get any hot water. I called the office and was told it had been turned off for the holiday and water would have to be heated up for the whole complex, which would take a few hours. Not having the time to wait, I showered and shaved with cold water and had started to get dressed when Dad turned up with the suits. We took what few of my things were left in the room and began the 30-minute drive. When we arrived, we could not find my wheelchair cushion. A wheelchair cushion is not an accessory, it is specially designed to aid posture and make sitting for long periods bearable. We think it had been left on the roof of the van as we drove away. There was no time to search for it, so we posed for a picture and made our way inside the church.

Seeing all our friends and relatives so happy for us did not make me nervous, I was looking forward to sharing the day with them. My dad and I took our positions at the end of the aisle and waited. I felt very safe and happy as I waited for Helen. The organist paused and then began the wedding march. Helen was a beautiful vision, slowly walking down the aisle with a kind of grace I was not used to. Her father looked proud as he walked with her. The ceremony went well, and passed by very quickly. We posed for pictures and people started to make their way to the reception – in the local pub where we had met seven years before. As we passed the war memorial in the churchyard, I felt a strong connection with the men on it, many of whom had also been married in the church. It was a hot summer's afternoon and we waited outside the marquee as our guests filed past, I began to feel nauseous after a while and had to find a bathroom. Out of the sun, I began to feel better and returned to the marquee. I had missed the meal, but I couldn't eat or drink anything anyway. The open bar was paid for by Helen's dad using money his mother had left when she passed away a few days before. A lot of our friends seemed the worse for wear; my friend, Dan, fell of his chair in mid-sentence. I read my speech and Helen, hers. Helen's speech had quite an opening. I still remember the silence that followed her opening joke: 'When I first met Richard, I thought he was a paedophile!'

We arrived at our hotel in Oxford that evening to find another wedding reception in full swing. We still had our wedding clothes on and Helen had a box with the last of my things from my room – mostly coat hangers. The receptionist asked us earnestly if a twin bedroom was OK. I looked at myself, then Helen, and shook my head. Back in another taxi, we were on our way to another hotel just outside Oxford where a bottle of champagne was waiting for us. The venue is now affectionately known as the 'Murder Hotel' as a guest was murdered there at a wedding in 2004.

We travelled by Eurostar the next day to Brussels for our honeymoon. We only had a weekend there. With its tiny medieval centre, dominated by European Parliament buildings, it was not the most romantic place I have been to. Feeling quite uncomfortable, we passed a mobility shop and were shocked at the price of a new gel cushion to replace the one my dad had lost. We ended up cutting the foam seat off an old office chair we found in a skip.

Using the computer in the hotel lobby, I learned that I had got a 2:1 in my degree, which was what I had hoped for. I graduated that summer, ten years after leaving school with almost no qualifications. I had worked very hard. I was also very proud to be the first member of my family ever to graduate from university. But I wasn't the last because Anthony and Mum graduated later.

OXFORD TO BIRMINGHAM

The transition into married life in our new home at Agnes Court was made easier by the fact that we had lived together at university. Although a newly built ground floor flat, it was, unadapted for a wheelchair user – the bathroom only had a bath in it, and I scalded myself pretty badly trying to use a rubber shower hose that fitted over the taps – but we made the best of it. Lively gospel singing, clapping and shouts of 'Amen!' and 'Tell it!' came from the neighbouring church every Sunday.

Slowly, the building filled with new tenants. The only couple we knew was in the flat next door. They had a new baby. As the post was dropped into a communal hallway, we soon noticed some of our post wasn't reaching us at all. We kept finding the communal front door open on the latch. I always made a point of shutting it properly. One morning, a note was taped to the front door asking for it to be kept open as a tenant had lost their key. Suspecting that we were one of a very few working couples in the building, we felt that we didn't belong there. Soon, things were being stolen, rubbish was lying around, written-off cars appeared in the parking spaces and the police were becoming regular visitors. One morning, we woke to see a mountain bike had been stolen and thrown over our fence onto our tiny patio. It was so sad to see a new environment falling apart. At the time, I was cross. I understand now that this was a valuable brush with poverty and that I had been conditioned to view my new neighbours with contempt and suspicion because they weren't like me. However, this was temporary accommodation; many of the tenants were from other cultures and were so poor and excluded from society that simply providing a nice building to live in was not enough to give them a sense of value in themselves.

My first job was a sabbatical position on the Students' Union Executive Committee at Oxford Brookes University. The wordy title was Deputy President: Welfare, Accommodation & Equal Opportunities. Working from the Students' Union Advice Centre, this was my first paid post and my first experience as a trustee. I undertook valuable National Union of Students training in 'running a charity' and 'effective representation and campaigning.' My new colleagues knew each other well already. In one session on working as a team, we answered aptitude questions about how we work. I emerged as a 'Plant', more of an ideas person and not a completer-finisher. Like a lazy horoscope prediction, this rang true enough, but it really bothered me for a long time until I eventually realised that this didn't have to be a binary judgement; being good at one thing doesn't necessarily make you bad at its opposite. It's about knowing yourself and being confident. True, I do start more things than I finish, but I am also thorough and do complete things. That is just how my process works – I need to have lots of ideas and only fully develop the best ones. Every team needs an ideas person!

As well as being a legally responsible trustee of the Students' Union charity and director of the Students' Union trading company, I represented the welfare needs of students to the university through numerous committees. I also organised and implemented large-scale welfare campaigns, set up and provided support for representative groups in the university's halls of residence, and worked in the Advice Centre.

Acting as a student representative, I was required to attend student disciplinary hearings. Sometimes it was hard to keep a straight face. In the first days of term, a drunk student rode an office chair down Headington Hill and crashed halfway down. The police were called. The university was concerned about its reputation. It was a moment of poor judgement on his part. I had to convince him that he did not want to fight the university on this and to apologise sincerely for putting his own and other people's lives at risk. Based in the Advice Centre, I was sometimes asked to speak to students as a former student myself. Often, students felt they were on the wrong course – on the course their parents wanted them to take, for example. I found that this was rarely a problem for students who had taken a gap year to find themselves before coming to university. I often wonder what Helen's life would be like if she had had taken a gap year. If she'd had the chance to get some distance from life at home and find herself, would she have still wanted me?

From my new office in the Students' Union Advice Centre, my first campaign was around mental health. I also held an alcohol-free night in a university building; it was a free event and open to all. I thought it might appeal to international students or those who didn't drink or just wanted a break from the intense alcohol culture. I printed and distributed flyers and put an advert in the Students' Union's paper, and bought a fair amount of soft drinks and sweets and music to play. Sadly, only a handful of people came. I think if I had put more work into it, made it a regular thing and provided entertainment on the first night, it might have fared better. As it was, it was an important lesson to learn. I never ran out of sweets or cans of pop for the rest of the year!

There was a lot of protesting on campus during this time. Tuition fees had been introduced in 1998 by Tony Blair's government; initially capped at £1,000, they have been increasing, along with the interest on the repayments, ever since. I went on a march in London with some Brookes students and, unable to meet up with them, I caught up with some of the reps from Oxford University. They introduced me to Sandi Toksvig. She was to stand as chancellor of Oxford University on an anti-tuition fees ticket. She shook my hand and said with a smile, 'You're tall enough to be on my netball team!'

Independently, we took to the streets again in February 2003 to protest against the war in Afghanistan. The column of people protesting in London was so long, I never saw the end of it. The diversity of the protesters was something. Young and old, male and female, Black and White, and disabled. It gave me hope that all these groups could come together for one another. I thought for sure that the voices of a million people could not be ignored, and was disappointed when the march wasn't given any coverage by the media. It struck me vividly then how the media can suppress popular opinion.

I deputised for the president halfway through that year, which engaged me in a more political role where I crossed paths with the university's chancellor, Jon Snow. At a formal dinner in Robert Maxwell's former home, the university offices in Headington, I introduced him to Helen. He said mysteriously: 'Well, of course I knew Richard before he was famous!' I have always puzzled about that. That year was a blur of networking and meeting new people. I was due to meet Charles Kennedy in London. He cancelled at the last minute for *personal reasons*. Who knows what could have happened if we had met! I did get to meet the Cheeky Girls, and their very formidable mother, when we booked them for one of our music nights.

One of our biggest achievements that year was the minibus. Despite its great success, its massive effect on student welfare, and my future as a bus man, I had nothing to do with it. Our savvy general secretary, Neil, had brought it to collect students from bars and clubs around Oxford and take them back to their halls of residence. Neil arranged all the permits, sponsorship, maintenance, and recruited the drivers.

At the end of this amazing year, I stood for re-election, and lost after a closely fought campaign and a recount. I left with a very strong belief in the principles of quality representation and the ethics of good public service. This fitted well with a career in local government, but it also disgusts me the way that many members of the current government behave.

We had been offered a couple of properties by the council. However, when we visited them, they proved to be completely unsuitable. Because I had specified ground-floor properties, I was being shown them all. They were usually in the housing estates of South-East Oxford and unadapted – in one, I couldn't get through the front door. In June 2003, we were offered a ground-floor flat in a troubled housing estate on the edge of Oxford. Although not in the areas we had specified, there were some good things about the flat in Blackbird Leys. All the windows were fitted with special levers and it had a small, shared garden with a raised flower bed. However, the bathroom had a bath and no shower, and there was only one bedroom. We had inherited this from the previous tenant who had everything set up to meet their specific needs. Before moving, I had to spend a day there letting contractors in. It was a hot sunny day and I hadn't brought anything to read, so I undressed and basked in the afternoon sun in the high-walled garden. Helen was appalled to find I had been sunbathing in the nude, and I had sunburn all over too. We set about making small changes to the flat. We were only there for six months.

I had a few months to find another job and was quite happy to stay within my comfort zone at the university. I applied for a few jobs there and with Oxford University, which I still thought needed to change. I also applied for a maternity cover job as part-time access officer at a district council in the south of Oxfordshire. Access officer was a new job title for me, but as the council's expert in disability, I was to act as an advocate, coordinator, and adviser for all access issues. I was excited to have another chance to make the world a better place! Relying on Helen to drop me off, I would arrive at my new office early every morning and I would go and read in the staff area. Abbey House was a modern-looking building.

Without air conditioning, it was uncomfortable in the hot summer months and cold in winter. The council also employed a tea lady, who would appear with a trolley full of snacks and offer tea and coffee. There were trips to council leisure centres and car parks. I worked with planners on the project to bring all of the council properties into compliance with the requirements of the Disability Discrimination Act, and developed and ran training sessions on disability awareness for council staff. I was eager to introduce them to the social model of disability. I enjoyed working with members of the public as I learned all about the physical aspects of access to and within buildings: ramps, doorways, corridors, lifts, showers, toilets, circulation, and evacuation.

I volunteered as a poll clerk for the council election in 2003. Uffington was a small, rural parish which was held by the Conservatives and was being challenged by Labour and Lib Dem candidates. There was a steady stream of voters at peak times. Some looked like they had come straight from the fields, their tractors still running in the car park. One asked, 'How do I vote BNP?' As poll clerk, I could tell him how to vote, but not how to vote for a particular party! I told him which logo was which so he could select one. He was disappointed that the BNP hadn't put a candidate up in the local elections. The seat stayed Conservative; the council was Liberal Democrat with a fifteen-seat majority. This election saw them lose four seats and stay in overall control.

In November, we were offered a purpose-built bungalow in Oxford with two bedrooms and a roll-in wet room. We even had our own garden. We had our laminate flooring moved from our previous place as it was still new. This dream home was wonderful; it also happened to be surrounded by aging council flats and newer social housing properties and suffered from the social problems common to these areas. We disturbed burglars within days of moving in. The police told us that our whole house had been ransacked. To our embarrassment, only the bedroom had been disturbed – the other rooms were just as we had left them (having just moved in). The burglars were not professionals who are only interested in cash, jewellery, and computer games. Although we had an alarm installed and tried to become part of the community, we always struggled to feel at home there. The bungalow bordered a footpath down one side and the local children played on our drive or on our roof. I felt that going to work was my only escape, so I found unemployment hard. We became friends with Simone and Mark, our neighbours. Simone already had four kids and was the same age as Helen. For all our differences, we all got on well. One night, Helen was invited to an Ann Summers party hosted by Simone. Later that evening, our doorbell rang, I answered it to find Simone in a sexy nun costume. Apparently, Helen had encouraged her to do it!

It was time to renew our Motability lease. Previously we had a Ford Focus Estate, which only

Helen was insured to drive. This time, we ordered a sporty four-door Focus with automatic transmission and hand controls. I had only had a few lessons in a bigger, higher car, so this was my first car, and I wanted to be the first to drive it. Still driving on my provisional license, I was determined to drive the car from the forecourt. It wasn't a very good decision. It was only 15 miles or so to Helen's tutoring job in Banbury, and it was over familiar road, but I was so tense that my touches were clumsy. I felt barely in control of the car, yet the sense of achievement that I was finally driving my own car and doing another thing that I had thought was impossible kept me focused on what I was doing. My instructor was a Black lady called Debra. She was direct; sometimes, her no-nonsense approach was difficult for me to work with. I panicked easily and had very low confidence. I put in a lot of practice with Helen, who helped me a lot with her kind, patient approach.

Fixed-term contracts were the way into local government for a lot of people. At the district council, mine was extended twice, and my hours increased to full-time. Despite moving me into a temporarily vacant post of equalities officer, the council eventually decided they could not find the funds to make my post permanent. At least I had some time to look for something else. With only a month in between, my next job was strategic policy officer, another fixed-term opportunity at Oxfordshire County Council. I applied for it because I wanted to work with more mainstream equalities issues, with better funding, and a higher profile. I was responsible for evaluating and improving the council's performance against the Equality Standard for Local Government and to carry out detailed work on individual policies and strategies. This included the council's new Transport Strategy. I had to highlight all issues with all groups using roads in Oxfordshire. This included pedestrians, cyclists, taxis and buses, and gave me a great insight into how everyone uses roads differently, but everyone depends on the road network. I also helped develop and implement a corporate Social Inclusion Strategy. I was able to run briefing sessions on this strategy for managers all over Oxfordshire.

In addition, I researched and wrote the authority's 'Guide to Culture and Faiths in Oxfordshire', a comprehensive guide for the fire and rescue service who would need to understand the customs of the people whose homes they were entering. As there were so many subgroups of the major ethnicities and religions that were identified in the 2001 Census as being active in Oxfordshire, it involved many meetings and much research. Thanks to my degree, I was comfortable with this. When I had compiled sections on each faith, I presented the guide to the council's multi-faith forum. A very competitive and argumentative group, each had edited their own sections, but one wanted to establish superiority over the others. The Jewish representative took me aside after the meeting and said: 'You must say that Christianity and

Islam are both beautiful daughters of Judaism, and this must be the first religion discussed.' I thanked her for her input, then explained that the guide was alphabetic for fairness and the introduction would be written by the deputy leader (I wrote it for him!).

Many of the other representatives were ministers. Talking to them helped me explore religion for myself. My favourite faith was Sikhism. I was impressed that their temples include a kitchen to feed the poor in their community. I also really enjoyed talking to the Humanist representative about living and dying. I do not believe in a God myself. We all have the power within ourselves to do good or evil things. I see organised religion as a man-made, external force. I admire people with a strong faith, and if the promise of reward or the fear of punishment motivates them to do good things – great. What I do not like is religions that seek to save you, or judge others. In *Small Gods* (Pratchett, 1992), Terry Pratchett sums it up for me when he writes: 'What have I always believed? That on the whole, and by and large, if a man lived properly, not according to what any priests said, but according to what seemed decent and honest inside, then it would, at the end, more or less, turn out all right.'

After all that, the 84-page guide was printed up and distributed through Oxfordshire. I was very fortunate to go on this journey of discovery. I also learned that Oxford and its county have a proud history of accepting refugees; from Spanish children during the Spanish Civil War, Jewish children during the Second World War, and Ukrainian families today. I appreciate that such an effort was a simple guide at best, closing with a very patronising list of do's and don'ts. It could never properly define the complexity of an individual, and so it was very much of its time. I hope it raised awareness. Much to my embarrassment, I had used the incorrect form of 'complement' when I said, 'this guide *compliments* the council's Race Equality Scheme.' I don't think anyone else noticed, until the deputy leader who put his name to the guide made it abundantly clear that he wasn't happy about it.

As I was still learning to drive, I would continue being dropped off for work early. In Oxford at 7am the only place open was a coffee shop. I would go in with a book and my iPod, and drink big mugs of double-strength coffee until it was time for work. Occasionally, I'd get trapped in their toilet because of the super heavy door.

It took me two attempts to pass my driving test. The first, I failed in the car park of the test centre. The instructor asked me to start the engine and drive forwards into the parking space in front. He then asked me to reverse into the space behind. I did it very slowly, checking my mirrors. I stopped the car and the instructor asked me if I had finished the manoeuvre. I replied that I had, and he scribbled furiously on his clipboard and we carried on. Little did I know that I already had a major fault. I had parked over two spaces; fallen leaves had covered the lines of the parking space I had backed into. We continued the test, which I thought went OK, but back at the test centre I was told I had not passed. I felt upset. Did the instructor not like me? Would I be doomed to fail my driving test for years like my mum? I retook the test in a few weeks' time and passed easily.

I drove Helen to work in Didcot at every opportunity before driving myself to work in Oxford. Hitting the city centre traffic with music playing in the car gave me such a powerful feeling. For ease of access, I was issued with a permit and a remote control to raise the barrier to the county council's tiny car park. I would park up and pull the wheels and frame over me from the passenger side, reconstruct the wheelchair outside the car, transfer into it, and go to work. My newfound freedom also meant I could go to a lot more matches at Villa Park. I took different people as my 'personal assistant'. They got a match ticket in return. For many, it was their first time pushing a wheelchair and it was interesting to see how the day played out depending on the part football, or drinking, played in their lives.

When I had been at the county council a few months, the team we shared the office with recruited a friend of mine from university. Gavin was the husband of the manager of the Advice Centre at the Students' Union. He was a big football fan and I enjoyed his company. When Wycombe Wanderers hosted Aston Villa in the FA Cup, a few of us from the office went along and were treated to an 8-3 match. I was hoping again for my contract to be made permanent and was assured it would be. But the political climate changed drastically as the council came under Conservative control following local elections.

Disenchanted with life on the Isle of Wight, my parents moved back to Oxfordshire, to a village near Banbury. They had enjoyed living on the island, until Mum had had a health scare and realised that the NHS there was not very good. My dad's new employer was sending him to the mainland every day anyway. Their new home was a bungalow with a converted loft. I welcomed the move because it was good to have your parents nearby and it had been difficult and expensive for us to visit them more than twice a year.

When I finished at the county council, my colleagues presented me with a cake, cards, and a generous collection. I had only been there a year. I had been lucky with my previous jobs since graduating: each of them were well paid. Unfortunately, all of them were twelve-month fixed-term opportunities. At first, I had been willing to take them to develop my skills and gain valuable experience in equality in the public sector, but now I felt ready for a full-time permanent post. As the post I was leaving was to be made permanent, my manager said that he felt confident that I would soon be back. I applied for it as soon as it was advertised. Then the new Tory leader of the county council declared in the press that he did not understand the post and did not feel it was necessary. The post quickly became a political football, a crusade for this Tory politician against bureaucracy and inefficiency, and a battle between officers and elected members. Members of the public were stopped in the street and asked on camera if they thought that a 50k social inclusion manager was necessary. The answer to such a one-sided question was a firm no. The 50k figure so often quoted was the total cost of the officer, including a salary. The issue dragged on painfully for some weeks, until eventually I received a letter from the council to say that the post had been withdrawn. The letter had not even been signed by anyone. I felt let down by the managers at the council who had promised the post would be continued. I also felt that all of my hard work had been devalued.

Another of this small-time politician's favourite windmills was political correctness, especially nomenclature. Nothing more than a bully, he would insist he was the 'chairman' of a meeting and that a chair was only a piece of furniture. It was thinly veiled misogyny, insisting that positions of leadership can only be held by a man, or someone identifying as a man. I knew my father-in-law, John, had had similar clashes over his refusal to follow this sexist convention. With him in mind, I left a meeting at this point and have never referred to myself as a chair*man*. But neither would I correct or shame anyone in a meeting for doing so themselves.

The importance of language

Let's define political correctness. Simply, it is modifying our language so as not to hurt others. Language is a living thing and constantly changes to represent groups who are throwing off centuries of discrimination. Minority groups may reclaim language that has oppressed them. Those words belong to them now and we should not use them. No one likes change or being corrected, but repeated use of such language shows our ignorance and is, quite rightly, a hate crime.

It makes me angry that we disabled people cannot choose the language other people use about us. This is a circular problem. The Disability Unit found that 34% of the general public felt unable to communicate meaningfully with a disabled person. Every February 28th, for example, is Rare Disease Day. That word: 'disease'. It grates on me. I don't like it at all. A disease is negative, contagious, unpleasant, and unwanted. Someone with a disease is broken and needs fixing. Fortunately, many people are now aware that it is an outdated term and saddles multiple people with very toxic labels. It simply fails to even come close to describing either ataxia or my complex relationship with it. I prefer 'condition', as this describes a neutral, changing state, something a person can actually live with. I have raised this with the gatekeepers of Rare Disease Day, who I imagine are not disabled themselves, to no avail. But how do we know which words to use? By hearing disabled voices in the media, listening and learning. The *Crip the Vote* movement emerged in 2016 as disability activists in the US sought to engage voters and encouraged politicians to have a national conversation about disability rights.

We are, or should be, accountable for the words we use. Unable to rely on knowing the 'correct' word, in this complex world of ours, we need to actually question why our words and our attitudes can hurt others.

Political correctness also draws attention to the inherent lack of respect for others that many people and politicians have. Treating minority groups with respect conflicts with the structure that has served their interests for hundreds of years. Men especially, have been able to say whatever they want and get away with it forever. They now have to cloak this discrimination and lash out bitterly when doing so. Right-wing media and politicians fuel a 'culture war' by evoking fictional enemies such as 'Liberal or metropolitan elites' or 'woke Leftists' to do so. They grossly simplify the principle of political correctness by saying things like 'you can't say anything anymore' or 'it's political correctness gone mad.'

Health and safety is another example of the introduction of procedures that have made our lives infinitely better but it is often used as a scapegoat by greedy employers whose attempts to exploit people are frustrated by it. 'It's health and safety gone mad.' This sense of outrage has also been picked up by the media and is used to condemn State interference. This short-sightedness and yearning for a simpler time was used by Brexiteers to sell a Brexit that would 'take back control.'

So, if we hear something that makes us feel uncomfortable, we should challenge it. This statement comes with a caveat! Don't belittle someone to do so. To issue an appropriate challenge, give the other person the benefit of the doubt, find a quiet moment and always look at their intention. Ask yourself, 'What is this person trying to say?' 'Is something being presumed?' 'How has this word developed?' You have to consider the context of the word and use your judgement. Then, with a solid foundation of understanding, we can try to explain our perspective – it is not difficult. This is how we learn from one another.

Arriving early for a recent engagement at the House of Commons, an MP went to all the trouble of leading us through endless corridors and security gates to where we needed to be. He then asked, 'So what happened to you then?' I knew he was not trying to cause offence, his senior background in the Armed Forces had given him a very direct approach. I knew I couldn't just leave it there so I wrote to him to thank him for his help, but also to gently remind him that it is rude to ask personal questions of disabled people. Learning that we have caused offence is uncomfortable because it forces us to own our choices and challenges our accepted version of society. Be mindful of the difference between public and personal information.

If you're not sure, ask. Surely if you ask someone's name, you remember it and don't keep getting it wrong.

When people aren't open to what you say, then it's time to move on. You cannot choose your family, you can build a family of friends, and expect them all to treat you and others with respect. If you do not challenge either ignorance or hate, you are colluding with it. Prejudices can be very deeply held and people do not appreciate being challenged. If you try to help and they just cannot understand, you do not need them in your life – let them go. I make mistakes, but I am willing to learn from them. I will not accept hate or ignorance from my friends in the same way as I do not accept such behaviour from public figures.

Out of work

With my contacts and reputation, I didn't think it would take me long to find another job. Certainly not ten months and another city. First, I applied for a scrutiny job at the county council, convinced I would be successful. The interview went well, but I did not get it. This started a long process of applying, going to interviews and getting rejected. I was convinced that the scheme that guarantees an interview for disabled people would give me an advantage, but I found that most employers did not understand the point of the scheme. They were pleased to interview disabled candidates, but didn't appreciate the financial support available or the benefit to all employees of an accessible workplace. Some were unwilling to take the risk and make an appointment.

I was playing the disability card a little because the competition for jobs was overwhelming. The job market in Oxford meant that between 50 and 100 people were applying for the same jobs as me. Jobs in equalities attract people from all sorts of backgrounds. Employers in Oxford had their pick of the most overqualified applicants imaginable. I'd imagine I was going up against Nobel Prize winners. As the equalities field is more developed in larger cities, I widened my search by applying for jobs in London and Birmingham. Originally from Birmingham myself, I have family there and had been going there regularly to watch football. Another plus was that going to interviews in London or Birmingham made me feel important. Wearing a suit and tie, and travelling on the train with commuters felt very positive. I was not worried about the journey or how I would find the offices, even how accessible they might or might not be. I really enjoyed my interview with the Disability Rights Commission in London, for instance. I felt that they were comfortable with disability. Actually, few other interview panels really impressed me.

Our savings were gone and I was receiving Job Seeker's Allowance (JSA) by Christmas. I was surprised to be still looking for work and began to wonder if I was applying for the right level of job. My target was a salary above the average graduate salary of 20k, which I thought was very modest, but I did apply for a few jobs below that. I soon learned that employers don't read applications, but scan them looking for something to exclude the candidate. For each, I had written 1,500 words of flowing prose about myself, my experience and its relevance to the post. I began to take a more concise approach, writing a paragraph under each point in the person specification to illustrate why I was the best candidate.

Another interview that stands out for me was at the Open University's regional office in Oxford. I felt I had a good chance as I had studied with them and had recently worked with Oxford Brookes. I arrived for the interview and began putting my chair together. When I opened the boot of the car, I found to my horror that I had left my footplates at home. There was no time to get them, so I carried on with the interview. I explained the problem, how it meant that I could not lift my feet from the ground while moving in my chair and would not be able to tour the building and grounds. I liked the interview panel and hoped that my show of courage and my passion would impress them enough to offer me the job. It didn't.

My father-in-law, John, told me about a vacancy in the Equalities Team at Brent Borough Council, where he was chief education officer. I applied. It was a very good salary and a long shot. I did not get shortlisted. I asked for feedback and was told I had not covered some of the points well enough, and although the panel felt that I had the necessary experience, I had not expressed it well enough in my application. The post was readvertised three months later and I applied again. This time I took care to ensure my application was bluntly functional and I was invited for assessment in London.

John took me with him to Brent and gave me lots of information to read before dropping me at the test centre. I was one of six candidates. As we introduced ourselves, it became clear that I was the only person from outside London, as well as the only White and visibly disabled person. I was used to being the only disabled person in a group, but coming to terms with race was a new challenge for me. For the assessors, we had to build a six-foot tower from materials provided. The other male candidate decided on his own project, building an elaborate base, for which one of the female candidates worked with him. As de facto leader, I organised everyone who was left to build a tower with me, encouraging them to work autonomously on whatever part they chose. It was a very loose arrangement, but it allowed everyone to shine. One of the other candidates wanted to show their awareness of the deadline by repeatedly asking me, 'How much time have we got left, Paul?' It was a good idea, just a shame she got my name wrong. Tower complete, I was pleased with our performance.

I drove in for the interview the following Monday, but got hopelessly lost on the North Circular. After an hour of driving around Outer London on a very hot day, I phoned John and he came to the rescue on his scooter. Very grateful for his help, I followed him back to Brent Town Hall and got to my interview with minutes to spare. I was invited back for a second interview and delivered a presentation. I didn't get the post; the panel felt my depth of knowledge was not current enough. To me, this was a result of not having worked with racial equality before and could be easily remedied. Adding to my disappointment, the job advert had stated that applications from males with a disability were being encouraged. When the chair of the panel told me that she felt equality posts were stepping stones for ambitious officers, it seemed like she was really an administrator and lacked commitment to equality work. As believing in what I do is important to me, I told myself that this was not the kind of person that I wanted to work for.

I had been looking for work for eight months when I applied for a very good post as an equality and diversity officer at Birmingham City Council – it was one of the highest paid jobs I had applied for. Mum was upset that we were even thinking of returning to Birmingham. She felt it was still the city she had left 30 years ago – the dark, dangerous place that my parents grew up in, saw changing, and did their best to leave. After not hearing anything for two months, I was invited to an interview. It was an intense two-day interview, which included psychometric testing, multiple panels, and exercises. I thought I'd represented myself well enough, which is the best you can hope for. As you have to when you are looking for work, I moved on and resumed applying for jobs. My JSA had finished and we were living off Helen's salary and my disability benefits. I had almost forgotten about the opportunity in Birmingham when, a month later, I was invited back for a second interview – this time with the head of diversity. Another month later, I received a letter offering me the post with a salary in the middle of the range advertised and explaining that I had been selected from nearly 100 other applicants.

My start date was Monday 2nd October, 2006, which would make it exactly one year since I had finished my last job. In the ten months I had been unemployed, I had applied for about 100 jobs and been to about 20 interviews. All of them were pebbles in the great stream of life that would have sent me in a completely different direction.

Back to Birmingham

I accepted, and we had two months to prepare for the move. Although going to Birmingham did not feel like a big step for me, I do regret being so selfish. Helen started looking for teaching posts in Birmingham while I concentrated on enjoying the summer and the World Cup! We also began looking for somewhere to live. My parents took us on a tour of Solihull, Olton, Knowle, and Shirley on the (acceptable) south side of the city. Nice, aspirational places that had been even nicer when my dad was working in the area some 25 years earlier. We wanted to move out of social housing and get onto the property ladder. We started a process of looking for a new home; completely unfamiliar with the whole process, we had a rough idea that we wanted to live in or around Solihull, and internet mortgage calculators told us we could borrow £220,000 on our combined salaries. Thank God we didn't need to. We found several ground-floor flats, and arranged to visit them over the summer. The flats varied in age, location and price. They were all too small. We decided this meant that we would only look at new builds. We found one that needed only minor alterations and were close to making an offer. I had sent emails to every social landlord in the region asking if they knew of or were building any accommodation for wheelchair users. The emails only provided dead ends until an agent of one of the landlords phoned me. They had some developments they thought we should look at. This was how we found a two-bedroom flat in a very nice area just outside Solihull, which was on offer on a shared ownership basis. We would buy a share of the flat and pay the landlord rent for theirs. Over time, we would pay the landlord off. I would be able to commute into Birmingham from Solihull or the NEC, which were both nearby.

We reserved the flat and began the process of getting a mortgage and arranging for the bathroom to be made accessible. With a deadline for moving by Christmas, I started my job and began the daily 165 mile-round trip by train. I would do this every day for the next three months. On my first day, Dad took a day off and came with me, getting on my train when it reached Banbury, meeting me for lunch, and coming back with me in the evening. This meant a lot.

I enjoyed the job; it was a new way of working for me. Birmingham City Council was huge, fast-moving and forward-thinking. I was part of a 52-member division that promoted equality and diversity across the entire council. I was attached to the Housing Department, helping managers to complete equality impact assessments on their services. In this way, I was now explaining equalities to managers who were keen to ensure their services were the most inclusive they could possibly be. I also coordinated monthly meetings of the Equality and Diversity Tenants' Group and produced the team's quarterly bulletin, as well as picking up some corporate work on disability. The tenants were interesting. This experience reminded me how equality work could limit your contact with actual people. The tenants were very suspicious of the council – for the first time in my career, this made me the enemy. I remember one angrily exclaiming, 'Next stop: Guantánamo Bay!' (the notorious internment camp set up in post-terrorist attack America where inmates were held without trial) when I asked for a few days to provide some information he had requested.

With a new job in new surroundings comes the chance to reinvent yourself. To take advantage of everything you have learned. For the first time in my life, I chose to present myself as professional and well-organised rather than the friendly, lovable office mascot. Like after my first day of secondary school, I decided to try and develop a harder edge. I was convinced that my new colleagues would be cutting-edge professionals and I would struggle to keep up. What I found were the same types of people I had worked with before, in the same proportions, but in greater numbers. I was shocked how dysfunctional the Equalities Division was. From what I could tell, at least a dozen people (some quite senior) were being paid without doing any real work. I had informal chats with concerned colleagues in my first week who all told me solemnly to 'keep my head down'. Sadly, there was as much manipulation and bullying going on as everywhere else I had worked. I was a little disappointed to find that I might have been appointed for my disability expertise as I had replaced the council's outspoken disability expert.

When I was not working, I was on the train on the phone with our bank, landlord, tradesmen who were installing a wet room in our new flat, or solicitor. Also, occasionally, eating or sleeping. I was keen to impress in my new job, so that added to the pressure I was under. It took me another hour to get to and from my office from New Street station. As I was there twice a day, I got to know the staff. The long commute was wearing me out. Despite my manager agreeing to my working from home one day a week, my health and relationship with Helen were under a lot of strain.

Where it had taken me months to get a job, Helen took just four days. With her Oxford degree and PGCE from Oxford Brooks, she was snapped up straight away by a comprehensive school on the edge of the city, a few miles from our new home. I felt that Helen had sold herself short and should have held out for a better school, but she liked the place, the children and the head of department, and preferred to work in a state school. Very grateful for her support, I didn't push it. She agreed to start in January.

We finally moved just days before Christmas 2006. Our new flat was in the social housing section of a wealthy development. The expensive cars owned by our neighbours placed us at the very bottom of the social hierarchy. With our own car park and an entrance tucked out of sight round the back of the building, I felt that we had gone from graduates with good, full-time jobs to 'scumbags'! Despite this, and with roots in Birmingham, and that lengthy commute behind me at last, I instantly felt at home in that cosmopolitan, bustling, young city. I felt we had made it through a very testing time together and looked forward to settling into our new home and new jobs. Our Christmas letter to friends and family echoed my optimism.

For our first Christmas in Birmingham, I received a copy of *Lucky Man* by Michael J. Fox (Fox, 2003) as a present. In the early stages of Parkinson's, his story of hard-won self-acceptance and optimism was a great influence on me. For those of you who don't know, Michael J. Fox was an icon of the 1980's. A talented actor with tremendous energy. He played the high-school time-traveller Marty McFly in the *Back to the Future* films. I was 15 when the saga was completed, and to me he was the cool older friend and mentor that everyone wanted to know or to be. He knew about girls, guitars, and how to stand up for yourself. Our lives have followed similar courses since then. Unknown to me, we went through similar traumas at roughly the same time. After an investigation of a twitching finger and a sore shoulder, Michael was diagnosed with early onset Parkinson's in 1991. At the same time, I was dealing with my diagnosis of Friedreich's ataxia. As I was 15 years younger, we were at different stages of our lives and faced different challenges. Michael was 30, married, with a 3-year-old son. It was the desolation of our bright futures that we both faced. I don't think we'd have been much help to each other if we had gone through it together! In 1998, he felt ready to go public with his condition. It had taken him seven years to come through the personal wilderness of his own diagnosis and it took me six. So, although we've never met, we share a special bond.

Much of his optimism for the future was channelled into the Michael J. Fox Foundation. The foundation has made a huge contribution to Parkinson's research, raising over two billion dollars, but as yet, as with my own condition, there is no cure. At the time, I didn't appreciate the importance of being involved in organisations that work to raise awareness of and find treatments for our conditions. This certainly influenced me to begin my own life-changing association with Ataxia UK.

As time marched on, I would see Michael appear occasionally on TV shows. He was a recurring character on *Curb Your Enthusiasm* as Larry David's neighbour, exploring stereotypes of disability and the awkwardness of people who just don't get it. He also appeared as a lawyer on *The Good Wife*, cynically using his disability in the courtroom to influence juries. In both, he appeared as himself. Physically shaking, his speech slurred and slightly slower, as he put extra effort into saying each word. Yet not afraid or ashamed of who he was. There would be the occasional buzz in the media from the excellent work of the foundation. His TV appearances became increasingly rare.

For me, his book was a reaffirmation of my own decisions to 'live for every day' and 'choose my friends carefully.' Most importantly, it reminded me that I was not alone in living with a progressive condition. Michael had searched his soul and confronted his future. He had stopped drinking and had come out fighting. Similar to my own life at that time, he was living with relatively few physical restrictions. He was still flying, taking family holidays, driving and working on film and TV, while acknowledging the difficult time ahead. He appreciated his family and made a time-traveller's promise to 'be more present.'

I was settling into my new commute from Solihull station to Snow Hill station, about half an hour altogether. I liked Snow Hill station; my grandfather used to work there when it was a busy freight depot. I got to know the staff at both stations a little more each day as they would wait with me on the platform with the ramp, ready to deploy it and send me off to or from Birmingham, or meet me when I got back. Lorna, one of the members of staff at Solihull station, made a sampler when my first child was born.

Within a couple of months of starting, I had a new manager. Peter was from Liverpool and had been with the council for some years. I had never worked with anyone like him before. Although seconded to the Housing Department, he had no respect for the head of diversity and focused on building links within the Housing Department. His approach to work was new to me. His infectious laugh, a mischievous chuckle, like Popeye's, would bounce around our open-plan office. Our team would sit together with tea and biscuits or food someone had brought from home and talk, sometimes for whole afternoons, and like a storyteller, he would tell his team about growing up as a young Black man in Liverpool or stories from his career. It reminded me of the conversations from *Desmond's*, Channel 4's early '90s sitcom about a Caribbean barbershop in Peckham that I loved to watch growing up. I loved the familiarity brought by the gently mocking rhetoric; always so powerful, also hilarious – the kind of way you would talk with your family. Peter's scouse wit worked well here. I'm sure others in our open-plan office would hear us laughing the afternoons away and wonder if we got any work done at all. But it wasn't idle gossip; he would skilfully link his stories to modern issues of race and culture. I felt accepted and learned more about equality and diversity and how racism works from him than any course I had been on.

Peter was close to retirement; his philosophy was that three years was about right before moving on and that the Equalities Division was nowhere to build a career. It was also difficult to leave such a specialised field. One colleague introduced me to the importance of career planning and to look for work outside my comfort zone. Luckily, Birmingham City Council was a massive organisation with plenty of opportunities for development.

At Easter, we took a much-needed break in Crete. It was our first ever adapted holiday. Instead of walking miles on our own, trips and transport were provided. Our hotel was next to a big German war cemetery, as Crete was the scene for the largest airborne invasion ever. We felt the islanders held British visitors in high regard thanks to the sacrifices made by British soldiers to defend the island. When we got back, we picked up our new Motability car. We had agreed to go back to an estate car, which would mean sacrificing some of my independence as I could not pass the frame of my chair through the narrower doors. The possibility of having children was raised and I was sad to say goodbye to my first car. Our new jobs meant we could afford some upgrades to our new one.

Going back to work after the summer break, Helen was struggling with her job. She started working later, attending meetings at short notice, and would leave me waiting at the train station with her phone switched off most evenings. Her manager would call her at home at the weekends to share her work problems. On top of her marking and preparation, the job was occupying most of her time. Sensing a problem, I suggested Helen ask for a meeting with her manager to discuss her workload, then one October morning, Helen came out of the shower crying. She never went back to that school.

Now it was time for me to help Helen. The doctor felt that her granny's recent death, the gradual cut in her medication for depression, the strain of looking after me, and stress at work were likely causes. Helen was put on a high dose of antidepressants. I was very worried about her; she had always walked a very fine line with her mental health, but was now distant and often threatened to kill me or herself in her very matter-of-fact way. This had reached such a precarious phase that the doctor told me it would be best to hide the bladed cutlery. My mum came and stayed with us, and I worked from home until Helen could be at home on her own.

I felt pretty powerless. I like fixing problems with action; I find it much harder to 'just live' with a problem. Unfortunately, clinical depression cannot be fixed. The strain of it all was becoming too much for me. Peter was very understanding. I was struggling with my own very superficial need for attention. Helen would go to bed between 8 and 9pm most nights, so I had a lot of empty time with no human contact. I caught up with friends online. One was in a difficult relationship herself and we enjoyed the attention we gave each other. She was there for me when I really needed someone to talk to.

I remembered how much our family pet, Dusty, had meant to me when I was at home alone all day doing my first courses with the Open University. I hoped that having a pet would be therapeutic for Helen, get her out of the house and into the fresh air, and that they could build a routine together. I also hoped that it might enable her to not depend on antidepressants in the long term and even help her prepare for motherhood. Helen's dad helped choose a breed. He had found a breeder of Irish Terriers in

Doncaster and Helen went to meet the puppies. She picked one and arranged to return to pick her up. We asked our landlord if it was OK to own a pet, as some of our well-to-do neighbours had, and were told that it was in our contract that we could not have pets. We challenged this and went to collect Tara as arranged. Over the next few weeks, we corresponded with our landlord. Our doctor even wrote on our behalf to say that a pet would enhance Helen's treatment for depression. Playing the disability card, we said that we intended to train her as a support dog for me. After two weeks of having an unauthorised pet in our flat, our landlord relented.

With the recovery going well, I booked flights to America and hired a car with hand controls so we could share the driving. I was hoping to recapture our early years of adventurous exploring together. We'd fly into San Francisco and out again from Las Vegas two weeks later. I had worked out an elaborate 2,000-mile itinerary that took us through the pine forests of Yosemite, Death Valley, down the Big Sur coastline, to LA, down to San Diego, the Grand Canyon and the Hoover Dam, to end in Las Vegas. We navigated coastal roads giving way to open desert highways by map. It felt quite daring to be living on fortune, not knowing where we were going to sleep each night.

The car I had requested was a convertible Ford Mustang, but the hand controls I needed could not be fitted to it, so we were offered a 'compact' car instead. When we collected it, there was nothing compact about this car, a crystal-blue Chevrolet Monte Carlo. Helen did most of the driving on those long, hot days, where the roof of the car was burning to the touch. Even the water we carried in the boot of the car would become too hot to drink. We were grateful the car had air-conditioning.

We worked well together and shared some great moments. We went panning for gold in a ghost town, drove along Nevada's extraterrestrial highway, and even crossed the border at Tijuana and went into Mexico. As we would only stop quite late on, dinner was often beer and wine we carried with us and snacks from the motel vending machines. One night, after a particularly long day of driving on a mostly empty highway, we were looking for somewhere to sleep. A brightly lit building duly appeared on the horizon. Relieved at the sight of this beacon of civilisation, I pronounced: 'We'll stop there.' As we got closer, we saw it was actually a gypsum refinery lit up so brightly as if it was on a flight path or to attract visitors from space.

Our hotel in Las Vegas had a roller coaster on the roof and we spent an evening in the casino. Unsurprisingly, in an environment designed to maximise customer expenditure (no clocks or daylight and free drinks brought to your seat), I was quickly spellbound by the flashing machines and fed in dollar after dollar. My free will gone, I was convinced the machine was just about to pay out. I was snapped back to reality by a spontaneous burst of applause at a nearby table. It was for Helen, who had just played a very good hand. She did extremely well at the blackjack table, covering my losses.

We had dinner in the Stratosphere rotating restaurant, the tallest observation tower in the US, right on the edge of the strip. Rotating once every eighty minutes, we could see the famous strip all lit up, and then the gloomy jumble of basic accommodation for the people who supported it stretching for miles into the distance behind. We had tickets to see the Cirque du Soleil – an erotic performance. Helen went to the bathroom during the first act and I got molested by a male performer in stockings and a basque who was roaming the audience with a microphone. We got matching tattoos in Las Vegas – a sea turtle with a green shell on our right shoulders. Helen went first, stoically locking her eyes on mine as the needle buzzed. I went second, playing it cool and not expecting much pain, but my sensitivity to pain must have changed. It took everything I had not to start crying and beg the guy to stop. In the years since, Helen says these tattoos link us as much as any ring or vow does. After coming back from America, Helen started cutting down on her medication and I noticed a change for the better almost straight away.

It was not plain sailing. On opening my lunch box one afternoon, my colleagues were very impressed that Helen had written a note for me. They thought it was romantic. In truth, it said, 'I hope you choke.' We all laughed and I explained that I had made a badly judged demand for some variety in my lunchtime sandwich fillings the day before.

I had felt for some time that the Equalities Division was being marginalised. Colleagues were leaving and not being replaced and the cabinet member for equalities made it clear that the whole division was under review and he would lead a restructure to make it 'fit for purpose'. The pay and grading system froze my salary. I felt that the head of diversity had done little to protect his staff. I didn't like the way I was used as the council's lead officer on disability when there was nothing about this in my job description. When I shared a proposal to start a network for disabled staff with the chief executive, I was told by the head of diversity that I had broken protocol by not coming to him first. He told me he was my boss and I should find another job if I didn't like it. I suddenly had no room for development. As mine was our only salary, I would have to look for another job much sooner than I had thought. The final warning for me was the head of equalities speaking at a conference. He explained that the division's task was coming to an end and he was looking for other areas to go into. I wrote 'I must move on now' in my notes.

In 2008, to prepare for the forthcoming inspection by the Audit Commission, Peter volunteered us to take part in the Housing Department's intense management assessment process. I emerged as the highest rated manager in my division. Following their inspection, the Audit Commission praised the department's Equality Impact Needs Assessment toolkit, designed to help managers integrate equality into their services on their own. It was a piece of work I had conducted alone. I knew I was an excellent manager, but wanted to show that there was much more to me than disability.

I applied for internal positions within the council, at the next grade up. I was invited to several interviews and was offered a post as a local housing manager within the Housing Department, managing a busy District Rent Team, annually collecting £4 million from about 10,000 homes (including tower blocks) in the North and later the Edgbaston districts of Birmingham. I managed the team's HR processes for twelve staff, conducting regular reviews and team meetings; I took the lead on areas of policy work and provided management support to colleagues across the council as required. As well as fulfilling the duties of the landlord for these tenants, I was responsible for providing strategic direction to ensure meeting targets for the recovery of rent arrears, checking legal papers to ensure the council met its duties as a landlord and made the final decisions in complex cases. I chaired tenancy reviews and attended tenant groups and the meetings of key area management colleagues. In the past, rent collectors would go door-to-door collecting rent and inspecting properties at will. Much of this interaction was now done electronically, with direct debits and by phone. The office was more like a call centre, with people wearing headsets and taking calls as they came through. I was expected to monitor the calls, soothe angry tenants, and help out if it was busy.

I was grateful to Peter for volunteering us to go through the Management Assessment Centre some months before. I had a mentor in a housing association and had been entered on the department's management course so I felt good about what I knew would be a big challenge for me. The Rent Division had been centralised into a modern building in the centre of Birmingham. I was sad to leave the Equality and Diversity Team – I felt I had done some very good work there. The great autonomy I had enjoyed in my work had helped me to do well. Before my 'free-transfer' to Birmingham City Council's Housing Department, the most important thing my new team wanted to know about their incoming boss was which football team he supported. We had a few departmental conferences in Villa Park's cavernous Holte Suite. I loved being there as much as some colleagues hated it! That's how important football is in Birmingham.

Helen and I took a break to Gran Canaria for a week to see our friend, Gary. As he was between jobs, he was able to stay in our apartment and share the holiday, showing us the side of life he knew there. We returned to Oxford to have tests to make sure that Helen did not carry the defective Friedreich's ataxia gene. The results came through a few weeks later: while our children would have a small chance of being carriers, they would definitely not have my condition. Just a little over a year after her breakdown, Helen had phased out her medication; we were in a strong relationship, had good jobs and a good network of support. We knew that we'd give our children a loving and happy childhood and bring them up to be exceptional people. Tara had played a huge part in Helen's recovery and we shared a huge attachment for our little dog. We decided we would try and start a family.

Finally out of the Equalities Division, I was feeling more settled at work, but the challenge of parenthood was about to be just as intense.

PARENTHOOD

I'd always wanted to have children ... we'd just never agreed exactly when. We all have some difficult choices to make to pursue this dream; we all have a choice. In our case, there were so many factors for us to consider. As human beings, we sometimes rely on our intuition and don't always make logical decisions. But there are no guarantees; none of us know what might happen. In life, we play the percentages, we assess the risks, look at what we can control and try to make our decisions accordingly. For someone with a disability, those percentages change considerably.

Dark thoughts can emerge too. I had focused on eugenics and medical killing during my degree, so was aware of the very worst things that the state and ordinary citizens can do to disabled people when they are dehumanised. I felt sad that, given my life expectancy, I would probably not know my children as adults. I feared they might become child carers, missing out on their childhood to care for an ailing parent. Perhaps they'd get bullied. I even wondered what kind of future they could look forward to in this terrible world.

Some things I was certain of. Firstly, I would not have wanted my parents to deny me a chance of life if they had had that choice before I was born. Secondly, that we must live for the moment. Thirdly, fear should not stop you but be seized as an opportunity to do great things.

Helen became pregnant in September 2008, and I started my new role as local housing manager in the November. I understood that a couple could expect to wait for anything up to a year to conceive, so I was surprised, and a little disappointed that it only took us two months. I bought Helen an ovulation kit which measures hormones and lets you know when you are ovulating. While I felt we still weren't trying hard enough, Helen says the conception was managed like a military exercise. She called me at work to let me know the news and I was shocked. I told my colleagues straight away and they shared my excitement.

Helen felt nauseous and tired for the first 12 weeks. As everything was fine in her 12-week scan, we went 'public' with our news. I proudly posted the pictures from the scan on Facebook. The 20-week scan came and went without a problem. I was relieved that there were no complications. Helen decided she wanted to know the sex of the baby if possible. The nurse was 85% sure it was a girl, which confirmed what both of us already felt. We had only really considered girls' names up to that point. Being shown around the delivery room in Solihull Hospital, the midwife showed us a CD player on a shelf in the corner and explained that partners often made a CD to play in labour – I understood from this that labour was no longer than a full-length CD, about an hour. I was very disturbed to find that anything up to 36 hours is more usual. I was pleased that our baby would be born a few miles from where I was born myself. Helen had had some hypnotherapy to ease her concerns about labour, and it seemed to have a positive effect on her general wellbeing. I don't know if it was the pregnancy or a combination of not having to work, or the hypnotherapy, but Helen seemed better than she ever had.

The baby kicked after Helen ate sweet food. Isn't that awe-inspiring? Being a prospective new parent opens a whole new world of behaviours, loads of baby equipment, and feelings. The sheer amount of equipment available is amazing. It is its own industry. I took a pragmatic approach to making sure we had all the essentials we needed when we needed it. By approach, I mean a spreadsheet. We were generously offered cots, toys, and clothes by friends. I began to feel great regret that I would probably not get to know my daughter, and would have to leave her in her early years and leave Helen alone to bring her up. Thoughts of this kind I had been able to suppress until then. I suppose every new parent has to face up to their own mortality. Each new child is a painful reminder that the circle of life has turned again and that we are not children ourselves any longer.

Much as Helen had decided when it was time to get married, she decided she was going to give birth about two weeks before the due date. She started having mild contractions on the Monday. I timed them throughout the day. There was not much I could do apart from be supportive and make sure Helen was eating and drinking to build up her strength. Helen found the TENS machine we had hired for pain relief via an electric current, helped. Gradually, the contractions lengthened and became more intense. We called the midwife who advised us to come in to the hospital. We took Helen's overnight bag and called a taxi. We arrived at teatime and were sent home again as Helen was only slightly dilated. We waited to see if there was any change. When there was not, we went home.

I got some sleep that night, but was up before sunrise timing the contractions again. The day proceeded as it had the day before. Helen was reluctant to go into the hospital again in case she was sent home. Around 7pm, Helen felt something move suddenly inside her, and it was time to go. We drove to the hospital, parked and made our way in. The doorway was partially blocked by a laundry wagon; we managed to squeeze past. Later, Helen told me she didn't think she was going to make it – to the hospital, or through the gap, I'm not sure. We arrived and were shown into the delivery suite with the birthing pool. After a quick examination, the midwife said Helen was fully dilated and too advanced to go in the pool. I put my CD on and waited, feeling helpless. The midwife said she thought the baby would arrive in two hours. My CD was too short.

The midwife broke the waters. The contractions were intense now, and Helen went on all fours to push. This went on for about four hours, four powerless hours from my perspective, until we could see the head – a mass of dark hair. I did not feel the rush of emotions I had expected; my concerns were for Helen. She was exhausted and her legs had gone to sleep so she stood next to the bed. I moved around to hold her hand; she gripped my arm tightly as she pushed. A doctor joined and helped Helen on the other side. The midwife was below, ready to catch. Helen would push and the top of the baby's head appeared, only to disappear as the push ended. After a few more pushes, the baby slid out into the arms of the midwife.

I had expected to fall deeply in love with our daughter as she arrived. The other fathers-to-be on our parenting course had agreed, but, instead, my main feelings were relief and hope that everything was OK with mother and baby. Exhausted, Helen laid back on the bed and our newborn daughter was laid on her chest. I was given some short scissors to cut the cord with. I remember the midwife was in the middle of telling me how tough some cords were to cut, as I handed her the scissors back, cord already cut. The baby was being cleaned, weighed, wrapped up, and put into my arms. She was a healthy girl, 8 lb 1 oz. I looked down; her face was flushed, and her tiny features were squashed due to the delivery. *She doesn't look much like me*, I thought, as I gave her back to the midwife. At this point, I wished I had moved back to the top end of the bed and stayed there. My advice to dads-to-be is: No matter what happens, stay at the head end!

Helen still had to deliver the placenta; the midwife waited as Helen wanted to deliver it naturally. Some time passed and nothing much happened. The doctor came back in and Helen was given an injection to bring on the delivery. The doctor hooked a tray under the end of the bed and gently pulled the placenta. It came out with a lot of dark blood and several large blood clots; the doctor began to sew, saying quite casually as she worked, 'The tearing is not too extensive; you have lost about a pint of blood and will need a few stitches.' I was absolutely terrified that she had lost so much blood. Without doubt, childbirth is a painful and traumatic experience for women. The powerlessness that partners go through should be recognised too. Stitching done, we were left alone as the midwife fetched us some tea and toast. Or perhaps that was just for my wife. It was about 2am. I texted our parents with the news and took a picture of

Bella in the cot. The circle of life continued; someone was giving birth in the next room and screaming like she was being murdered.

After her tea and toast, I encouraged Helen to cross the room to see Bella. My mistake. After a few steps, she went pale and crumpled to the floor. Her eyes never left mine as she lost consciousness. I called for help and a team of nurses came into the room and helped Helen back into bed. We were left alone again. Soon Helen needed to go to the toilet – it was an en-suite. To be on the safe side, we asked a nurse to help. It was on the way back to the bed that she collapsed again. After waiting for the results of a blood test, Helen was given a saline drip and moved upstairs to the ward to rest. I thought she should have a blood transfusion, which didn't happen for a few days. I went for breakfast in the hospital canteen and sent more texts. I was scared and exhausted; I took a taxi home and went straight to bed. I would be back at the hospital later that day. I returned with John and Sue. Helen was in a ward with several other new mums. She needed to stay overnight as the iron levels in her blood were too low. The next day, Helen finally had a blood transfusion and had to stay that night too. Helen was able to come home the next day.

The first few days did not go so well. The surface of our nursery chest of drawers doubled as a changing surface. When Helen was changing Bella, she rolled off it and fell into a plastic bin. Her crying only lasted a minute and she seemed fine. We decided to do the right thing anyway and take her to hospital to get checked, as a precaution. Because of our medical histories, this selfless action by two naïve new parents ended up with a case conference involving social workers and the police, which imposed a series of home visits on us over the next few months. I would work from home whenever these visits took place to support Helen, who found them very stressful. I understand that the authorities cannot take chances when it comes to child welfare, but it was clear that we were good people and were no threat to our daughter's safety. We were both made to feel that we were unfit parents and only changed Bella on the floor after that.

Back at work after two weeks of parental leave, I soon realised that what had always been important to me – work – was suddenly not so important now and it was stopping me spending time at home with Helen and our daughter. I missed them terribly. We also needed a home with a garden and a bit more space. I had heard that Bourneville Village Trust was developing some new accessible homes, so I enquired. We went to see a finished phase one home, which looked great. Our new home would be a three-bedroom house in the Selly Oak area of Birmingham with an adapted kitchen, lift and garden. The first step was to sell our flat. As it was shared ownership, we had to find a buyer for our share and have enough left over to pay the rent.

Although this was supposed to be a positive move

for us, Helen was very anxious from our very first night in our new home: the traffic noise from the main road was too loud, and she felt isolated from friends and family. Helen was unhappy. Wrongly thinking it was about me, I decided her unhappiness was because she was convinced that she would need to be nearer her parents to look after me in the future. I became upset. We argued a lot and I discovered that she had been looking at properties in Oxfordshire with her parents without me knowing.

As the homes around us were finished, people began to arrive. Our new neighbours were a young Sikh couple, Sunny and Kalvinder. We spent a lot of time helping them with job applications or benefit claims and they welcomed us into their dramatic lives. Sunny was a traditional Sikh drummer, so we would often hear him practising.

Now that we lived on a bus route, I could catch the bus into town every morning. The route was interesting, as we would start in Weoley Castle. It was pretty rough there. Passengers often got on there with strong body odour, facial tattoos, and what looked to me like attack dogs but were probably beloved family pets. It got gradually nicer as we went through the suburbs of Harborne and Edgbaston, gradually collecting more commuters like me, down to our stop at the end of Broad Street. If a bus broke down, the next bus was only 30 minutes behind. Drivers were generally OK, but occasionally you'd get one who was unhelpful or reluctant to move from his cab to deploy the ramp, especially in bad weather. The engine had to be switched off for the ramp to be deployed, and there was always a heart-stopping moment as the engine restarted after I was on board. I enjoyed travelling on the bus. I would listen to the *Adam and Joe* radio show with my headphones in, startling the other passengers by randomly laughing out loud. When Bella started walking, her and Helen would come with me to the bus stop on our street in the mornings. I would watch her toddling back slowly and carefully, holding her mummy's hand, and it broke my heart to leave them.

Work was challenging too. Whereas in previous jobs I had been something of a champion of outsiders, I now felt like I was 'the man', chasing them for rent and evicting them 'for their own good'. Working with tenants in rent arrears was difficult. Trapped in cycles of poverty, abuse, crime, poor health or drug use, there was little chance they would be able to turn their fortunes around. Christmas evictions were always hardest. Like Scrooge, I'd sign the warrant and housing officer and bailiff would enter, not knowing what to expect and to change the locks. The officer had to photograph every room and I had to review each set. The squalor was unbelievable. Evidence of children, broken toys or a brightly coloured bedspread, was especially heart-breaking.

I would tell myself that these tenants were hopeless, lacking pride or moral fibre and evicted themselves. Nicely blaming the situation on them and not making me a part of the problem. But I remembered living in temporary accommodation myself, and how little people in poverty have to live on. The problem of rent arrears is so much bigger than a lack of personal responsibility: it is poverty. Thatcher presided over the sale of the nicest council homes in the '80s and they were never replaced. The council tenants needed holistic support, not me lecturing them at a tenancy review, if they ever turned up, on the importance of maintaining their tenancy. Only a massive increase of affordable housing, a supportive benefits system and properly funded public services can free tenants from the constraints of poverty. If poverty is tackled, rent arrears and many other social problems would disappear overnight.

The housing officers in my team had been set up to work remotely with one day a week in the office. Because I was office based, I had to ask for it. It still felt like a grudging concession to a disabled employee. It wasn't too difficult to set me up to work for two days a month at home; I just had to fill a form in showing tasks completed and time spent on them. I found that, as a manager, there was unwelcome pressure on me to conform. I had always been a member of Unison throughout my career, serving as an officer when I worked at Oxfordshire County Council. Birmingham City Council was in turmoil. There were constant restructures, requests for voluntary redundancy and widespread fire and rehire. Unison had called a strike. I readily agreed and informed my bosses that I would be striking. I was summoned, alone, to a meeting with my manager and was made to feel like I was letting my colleagues down and that I was marking myself out as an enemy of the council. I was asked to reconsider. Recall that I knew from my experience of McDonald's to be wary of people with a bit of power trying to make me feel guilty for doing the right thing. I had to trust my instincts. I repeated my intention to withdraw my labour. I wasn't letting my colleagues down, I was representing them. Then, on the day before the strike, it was called off. I was proud that I'd stuck to my principles and a little cross that I hadn't been able to join the picket line. Starved of funding, Birmingham City Council eventually declared itself bankrupt in 2023.

I can always be relied upon to think of things in a slightly different way. For example, in quite a high-level departmental meeting, my fellow managers and I were asked how the alcohol handwash provided by the council during the swine flu epidemic (remember that one?) had gone down with our staff. With lightning speed, I replied that, 'It was OK, but you can't make a decent margarita out of it.' My comment barely registered a smile amongst my colleagues. Maybe I hadn't 'read the room.' It is still one of my favourite stories because it portrays me as quick-witted – a quality I admire in others and rarely exhibit myself. I'm pretty sure that it happened like that; to be honest, it is difficult to know where the truth ends and the story begins anymore!

I had just completed my third year at the Rent Division. I was proud that I was finally doing a job outside of my expertise on equalities, but there was little satisfaction to be found in the position itself. As we worked in a modern building with air-conditioning, I had never had so many throat infections. My chair picked up static that would discharge painfully with a loud crack whenever I touched the lift – giving me a lasting aversion to pressing lift buttons. Full-time work was becoming too much for me. I just didn't realise how much ... you never do until something happens.

CONCLUSION: A DAY IN THE LIFE

Having a successful, traditional career was one of my measures of success. I really enjoyed the social element of work. Being part of something bigger than myself and setting a positive example to others was (and still is) important to me. It was great for building my self-confidence and self-esteem.

I was also fortunate to work in local government. It fitted with my newly found sense of public service and came with the approval of Helen's parents. A YouGov poll published in 2020 on work/life balance found that 82% of workers in the public sector found their jobs to be meaningful compared to 64% of private sector workers. I developed many useful skills, and the pension scheme and the salary were great. I had learned a lot about disability, equality, and had several brushes with poverty. As an access officer, I had learned about the physical side of access, and my work as a policy officer showed me that inclusive services depend just as much on accessible procedures.

In my twelve months of unemployment, I had found a new level of determination in myself. I had borne so many rejections. In the end it had taken me over a hundred applications, some for jobs in London and Birmingham, to find my next job. I never gave up. A thing about applying for jobs is the mental contortions you have to put yourself through. As you apply for each job, you have to convince yourself that it is a perfect match for you. You must increase this for an interview, believing that this job will mean a new life for you. When the rejection comes, you have to readjust your thinking to 'it wasn't the right job for me' and find reasons why you have had a lucky escape. I don't think this manipulation is good for mental health, but you have no choice. You cannot afford to be bitter or give up. Applying for jobs needs to be done continually. So, while you're waiting for an interview, you need to be applying for more jobs, convincing yourself that this one is the job for you as well.

I had developed formidable resilience. I arrived at my first jobs hours early and relied on public transport when living in Birmingham, and I especially remember the gruelling 5-hour round trip from Oxford to Birmingham I made for the first few months I worked there. Trying to make good things happen, I tirelessly sought to improve our housing situation.

From then on, working in the Equalities Division

Conclusion: A Day in the Life

at Birmingham City Council showed me the national and historical contexts of equality in the UK, and I developed quite an expertise for explaining equalities to others. I learned that you have to make sacrifices to be successful, but a shortcut to success is to unleash your narcissistic personality and be prepared to 'stamp on other people.' Power always attracts bullies and they're never really happy. Working in the public sector meant that such careerists were the exception, and I could flourish. No matter how well liked you are, standing still is not an option. Planning and personal development is essential; however, I realised what was most important to me. Without knowing, I had developed my own work ethic: work hard, be kind, and keep moving.

Becoming a parent changes everything. There is a whole new world of responsibilities and feelings. There are sacrifices, grey hair and a lot of graft. To balance this out, such amazing and wonderful things happen when you're a parent. There are the birthdays, the first words, the first steps, the first day of school, the nativities, the sports days, Christmases. Children are a pure light that shine on you, on everything and everyone else.

One thing I didn't realise is that, although they recognise you, children don't start making memories until about four; all those sleepless nights, expensive family holidays, bedtime stories – they won't remember them! Spare a thought for your own parents and take lots of pictures! Being a dad is the best thing I've ever done; our children make me proud every day and it is a privilege for me to know them. I stand by the choice we made to bring them into this world. I hope they will look back when they're older and agree it was a good one.

I worked full-time throughout and made the all-important leap to a well-paid job that did not directly require my disability expertise. My time in the Rent Service proved I was a good manager, passionate about supporting others, and that a lot of people were purposefully trapped in cycles of poverty they could never get out of. I had finally become Nietzsche's Übermensch (superman). I had followed my own will to power, overcame myself and achieved excellence. I still didn't have the most important aspect of being a superhero; a cause to fight for or against. I had learned so much and had enjoyed working, but now working full-time just wasn't working for me. Without noticing, it had become a treadmill. I felt constant pressure to prove myself, to not have time off sick and stay longer at the office. I skipped too many lunches and ate too many takeaways. Tiredness had dogged me throughout my career; now it was getting too much for me. I had started to banish Helen to the spare room so I could grasp some peaceful sleep. Parenthood showed me how time-poor I was; I just wasn't around as much as I wanted to be for our daughter's early years. 'Chasing normal' was damaging all of us. Something had to give.

Part Four

(Just Like) Starting Over

I knew that full-time work was no longer right for me and I desperately wanted out. My hope now was to wind down gradually over the next six months and find a part-time role before enduring another office move/restructure.

THE NEW LIFE

When my manager told me that reducing my hours was not possible, I wondered if this was due to my union involvement. I also knew that this was discriminatory and that I would need the support of a more senior authority, so I asked to be referred to the council's Occupational Health Department.

This is how disabled people have been minimalised for generations. What do I mean? Another way of seeing disability is known as the medical model of disability. The opposite of the social model of disability, the medical model places guilt and shame on the disabled person. It is perpetuated by society, strengthened by our institutions and, as the name suggests, often held by medical professionals. Unable to conform to the widely accepted 'norm', a disabled person is framed as a 'tragic victim of cruel misfortune'; they are given the 'sick role' and excluded from mainstream society. Deemed unable to work, have families or live independently, they are denied many basic human rights and become the responsibility of medical professionals until such time as they are 'cured'. This leads to the segregation, infantilism and desexualisation of disabled people. This was to be the only time that I benefitted from being perceived as 'sick' by a medical professional.

Some close relatives of the medical model are the charitable and the biopsychosocial model. The charitable model individualises disability again but seeks to 'help' disabled people by generating pity for them. An example is the telethons that still dominate the fundraising world. The biopsychosocial model, developed through the private healthcare system in the US, can be seen in the UK benefit system's obsession with fitness for work. Access to benefits are assessed on what a person can't do, not what they can. Many charities report that people with terminal illnesses have been judged fit for by the Department for Work and Pensions (DWP).

This dilemma catches many disabled people out when applying for benefits they are entitled to. Rightly, disabled people want to focus on what they can do and not be defined by their disability. Unfortunately, the usually underqualified DWP assessors only award points for what claimants can't do. In 2015, the suicides of 600 claimants were linked to the DWP's assessment system over the previous three years. Since the government's transfer of people from the Disability Living Allowance to the Personal Independence Payment, Disability Rights UK report (Disability Rights Commission, 2020) that over 100,000 disabled people have lost their mobility vehicles and a further 200,000 who used their mobility allowance to cover taxis or general care needs to live independently have lost that too. This is an absolute disgrace and shows how badly our society needs to reconsider disability.

Back to the doctor assessing my status. He asked a few questions, which I answered honestly. I was looking for his agreement that I should reduce my hours and hadn't expected his surprise that I was still working at all. He said, 'You should have retired years ago.' It was such a relief to have someone tell me that I should stop. Outside, in shock, I phoned Helen. She listened and responded by angrily asking, 'What will we do for income?' and 'I suppose that means I'll have to get a job.' A practical response.

The next day, I told my team. Some admitted they were relieved as they had been concerned about my health for months. I was disappointed that they hadn't been able to tell me this, and that neither I nor Helen had noticed how much of a struggle working full-time had become for me. Once I got over the initial shock, I accepted that retiring was the right thing to do. I stopped work on 11 November 2011 and was officially signed off sick with 'physical tiredness.' Is there another kind? I applied for ill-health retirement and awaited the process: a report from my GP, another appointment with the council doctor, forms signed by myself and my manager, further evidence from my medical notes, a review by an independent doctor and a final decision by the pension company's doctor. Easy! The process took many months, partly due to unbearable slowness on my manager's part. A shame, because I always aimed to complete admin tasks for my staff as quickly as I could. Ill-health retirement meant that I became eligible for my pension and it was paid as if I had reached my proper retirement age of 65. It also meant that Helen would receive a payment for life if anything happened to me.

At just 35, I was suddenly facing retirement. I had worked with colleagues who had taken voluntary redundancy and knew it was a huge step, and that years of planning usually went into retirement. It's a big shock; your income changes and so does your status in life. Settling back into the family routine is a challenge. It was for me – everyone else, even the dog, was now higher than me in the pecking order. Remembering how courses with the Open University had filled my time while Helen was at university, I took the opportunity to continue my studies and to develop my writing. I started a Creative Writing Course. I was provided with a laptop and dictation software, which I found quite useful for editing. Dictating is a skill, as in you need to have an idea of what you want to say before dictating it. When I write, I only end up keeping about 10% of what I have originally written. I get the ideas down first, then have to develop them – a lot. The course started with a warning that writing draws on personal experience and we needed to be careful who we shared our coursework with.

I learned about how I wrote, and techniques to enhance it. Experimenting with new genres such as a screenplay or a sonnet was fun. A bit like an old deck of tarot cards, certain characters and themes recurred and became comfortable for me as I explored them – the courtesan, the leader, death, and the sociopath. I was able to explore aspects of my own personality through them, such as loss, isolation, broken relationships, unhappiness and redemption. As a graduate in Modern History, wartime was a common setting too. You may have noticed that there is also a little humour in my writing?

Tara, the life-saving terrier

Now it was time for our dog to save my life. We noticed that Tara responded quite strongly when anyone was in distress – this was usually me. Sure, she would helpfully bring a shoe, lick my face, or bark at me if I had fallen out of my wheelchair. Probably not what you really want when lying on a cold floor. Could we train her to develop this reaction? We had thought about it when she was a puppy, but decided against sending our beloved pet away to be trained. We were so excited when we learned that Dog A.I.D., a local charity, worked with people to train their pets at home. Even though the charity didn't usually work with adult dogs, the fact that Helen had already trained Tara to a very high standard tipped the balance for us. As I had so much time to fill, I was to take responsibility for her training. Being a terrier, food was everything to Tara and I spent the next year adjusting to life at home with a bag full of chopped cheese on me at all times.

After a year of intense training, Tara could retrieve (non-edible) dropped items for me, jump to switch light switches on, and bark fiercely at the doorbell or if I was in distress. Expectantly, people would ask me what 'tricks' she could do for me. I would reply, 'We trained her to answer the phone, but nobody could understand her!' Often people didn't find that funny. Perhaps they weren't expecting a silly answer to a serious question or were disappointed that Tara didn't help me get dressed or balance the household finances. I was trying to show that they were missing the point.

Beyond these 'tricks', what Tara really did for me was quite unexpected. She restored my link with humanity. If I was out and about in my wheelchair, people would look straight through me. When I was with Tara, it was like being with a film star. Suddenly, we were surrounded with people asking about her. We even had traffic stop on a busy road so one driver could get out of their car and say hello to us. I never realised this was something a support dog could do. It is so important for anyone who finds themselves at the edge of society to continue to interact with others.

Helen and I had agreed we no longer had a strong reason to stay in Birmingham so she had been looking at properties near her parents. Although I was reluctant to leave our purpose-built home, I wanted Helen to be happy and didn't want her to have to stay in Birmingham after she had moved there to support me and had such a difficult time. I joked that Warwick or maybe Leamington was the closest I wanted us to be to her parents, but as we had agreed we would talk about having another child once we moved, I think Helen was looking forward to the extra support we would get from living closer to her parents. We went to a few viewings in their locality. Nothing 'jumped out' and I was uncomfortable applying for a mortgage before my retirement pension was confirmed.

Driving had always been important to me, but it was very demanding. I had managed ten years, until the amount of time I could drive for began decreasing. I avoided night driving, especially on country roads. Not possessing the wisdom to know when to stop driving, One time I turned into oncoming traffic at a junction without checking properly. Helen, Bella and Tara were in the car and were all ok, despite both airbags being deployed in a shower of burning powder. I won't forget awkwardly having to explain to a passer-by who checked I was OK that I couldn't get out of my car without my wheelchair, or waiting for the recovery vehicle with Bella still in her car seat on the pavement next to us. Despite the low speeds involved, our car was a write-off. I never drove again.

Almost a year later, my pension was finally confirmed and I bought a THERA-Trainer exercise machine through instalments. It's an exercise bike with a motor connected to the pedals and hand cranks to assist you. It's very heavy. I had tried one before at a rehabilitation centre in Birmingham and was so impressed I knew I had to get one! I strap myself in and use it for an hour every day. I'm sure it improves my digestion, cardio, muscle mass, and circulation. It is in front of the TV, so I use it whilst watching in the evenings. I do feel my muscles tighten if I cannot use it for a few days.

The freedom of retirement showed me that I had spent the last ten years ticking boxes. Boxes that were not mine. I had become so focused on working, I needed to be told when to let go. Then I had a eureka moment: through volunteering, I hoped I could use my free time, utilise my skills, make a real difference, and find my own boxes to tick.

A New Home

Continuing my studies with the Open University and becoming a dog trainer filled some of my time, but I was longing for a challenge. Influenced by the strength that Michael J. Fox drew from his work with his foundation, I finally got involved with the charity that represents people with my own condition, the one I had stubbornly stayed well away from for twenty years, Ataxia UK. I had skills and experience that I knew would be useful. With support from Ataxia UK, a friend and I set up and ran its Birmingham branch. I gave an awareness-raising presentation on ataxia to a group of trainee physiotherapists at a hospital in Halesowen, and Ataxia UK chose the Birmingham branch as one of the areas they would run an awareness campaign in. I went to meet Millie-May, the young star of our campaign, and her mum. I started going to Ataxia UK's National Conference, which my brother, Anthony, had been enjoying for a few years. For quite a while, other delegates would look at me blankly until I mentioned him. 'Oh, you're Ant's brother.' After a few years of this, I started replying, 'No, he's *my* brother.'

Helen found a bungalow in a West Oxfordshire village. It needed a lot of updating, but had potential in bucketloads. We had to have it. The village was only a few miles away from where we met. Two of our friends lived there – we had been to their wedding reception there and often visited them. Middle Barton is bigger than Barford St Michael, with a shop, two pubs, a primary school, a members' club, and a village hall. One of the pubs was trading as an Indian restaurant and I was delighted to find the food was of a good standard. At least I would still be able to get a decent curry!

The remodelling and extension of our bungalow was down to our brother-in-law, Tom, a gifted architect. He planned and coordinated all the work. All the doorways were widened, the house was rewired, and underfloor heating was laid in the kitchen and extension. The extension was a high, open space which incorporates the sides of the roof above and a cast-iron wood burning stove (in case of the apocalypse) at the far end. On one side – and replacing the old garage – was a large bedroom with an en-suite wet-room. We had the ceiling reinforced so we could support the addition of a ceiling track for a hoist. The room was finished with a large American ceiling fan, gifted to us by my dad as a housewarming present. With our slightly lowered ceiling, it seemed to dominate the room. Helen requested it be fitted above where I lie in bed, so that if it dropped off, it would only maim me. I don't know if she was joking! She was very grateful for it when pregnant with Billy and every hot summer since. The extension is an impressive space; I've been happy to hold some important meetings and poker games there.

Adjusting to life in a small village was a challenge at first. In Birmingham, I would feel quite anonymous as a wheelchair user, but in a village where everyone knows everyone else, I knew I would be an exceptional sight. When we were introducing ourselves around the village, we were struck by how everyone seemed to know the full history of our house and its previous occupants. 'Ooh, you're next door to Anne Marie!' quite a few people would exclaim in a hushed, conspiratorial tone. I was worried that we had moved in next to a Bond-style supervillain or cat lady – I was hoping for Catwoman! It reminded me of an incident years ago when Helen and I were on a holiday in deepest Norfolk. I had parked in a large pub car park and we had just swapped over as drivers, and bumped another parked car as we turned around. We could not see any damage and it was quite a battered car anyway. We were just going to leave a note when somebody came up to us, sucked in their breath and said: 'Oh, that's Alan's car' with a pained expression and a slow shake of the head. Like he was some kind of monster, or we had murdered poor Alan. 'I'd better go and get him.' We waited to see who or what would emerge from the pub and how angry he would be. When he did come out, he wasn't a Shrek but was obviously a beloved, elderly local. He couldn't see any damage and wished us luck on the rest of our journey. Similarly, Anne Marie turned out to be a popular mum that everyone in the village knew, showing that first impressions are important and should never be rushed.

Finding Ataxia UK

A life-changing moment for me was when I first joined Ataxia UK's Board of Trustees in April 2013. It was one of those pebbles in the stream of life that changed my direction forever. I say first, because I had to step down a month later.

Having started my career as a trustee of the

Oxford Brookes Students' Union, I knew something of running a company with great people who had powerful motivations and who brought unique skills and experiences with them. I applied for a grant from Ataxia UK to go towards the adaptations in our new kitchen. It would feature lowered worktops, a sink, and an induction hob. As a new trustee, this made some of my fellow trustees feel uncomfortable. I felt that as a person with ataxia, it was acceptable for me to take a role in running the charity and still apply to access funds available to all of its members. I did not expect nor receive special consideration. Some of the board, mostly people with relatives with ataxia, threatened to resign over it. Under pressure, I stepped down from my trustee role for the next six months, but it had awakened in me the simple idea that Ataxia UK had to be run by and for people with ataxia.

I rejoined Ataxia UK's board in October 2013. There had been movement in my absence and there was to be a new incoming chair. Dr Harriet Brown was a kind and supportive chair for much of my time as a trustee, plus the most organised person I've ever met. The same age as me, Harriet had also taken medical retirement at the same time as me. For those reasons, we often joked about being twins. Difficulties with her hearing meant that Harriet used a stenographer to follow conversations around the boardroom. Her example showed me that Ataxia UK could be well run by people with ataxia.

My early days as a trustee were more passive, receiving reports and accounts and developing strategy. As my confidence grew, I felt able to get involved more. I found the time spent with other trustees as we drove to meetings or conferences to be invaluable. I found that you got to know more about your fellow trustees by spending a couple of hours with them in a car than you did in a few years of board meetings. A very good friend I made this way is Andy Downie. He has a son my age with Friedreich's ataxia and can spot a circular argument from a mile away. I also got to work with members of staff who are some of the best in their fields.

I began another course with the Open University: Advanced Creative Writing. This time, the tutorials were in Summertown, Oxford. The course focused on a deeper exploration of techniques, which for me underlined the importance of having others look at your work and comment through an online forum. Such feedback can change the direction of a piece of work and would later encourage me to share stories I had written on my blog.

Once we had settled in to our new home, new and interesting volunteering opportunities seemed to find me and my time began to fill up. I often tell people that I am busier now than when I was working full-time! While my volunteering portfolio became much more fulfilling, each opportunity dovetailed nicely into the others.

I fulfilled my dream of being a superhero's

sidekick. Just after we moved to Oxfordshire, I returned to Birmingham to complete the Birmingham half marathon with a friend. He was going to push me around the course in my chair – I was happy to be of assistance to his self-torture. We tried to coordinate our outfits over the phone. Mark wanted us to be the dynamic duo and already had a Batman costume. I agreed to dress up as Robin. When we met up on the day of the marathon, Mark – a big, fit guy – was wearing a '90s homoerotic batman costume complete with bulging muscles, and I was wearing a '60s Robin outfit complete with green tights. I wish I checked which era Batman he was coming as. As we rattled around the streets of central Birmingham, I felt every bump. We were going too fast, but Mark reprimanded me whenever I gripped my push rims to slow down. Knowing that a pothole could eject me from my chair at any moment, I just hung on for dear life. Spectators would instantly recognise Mark's character and call out, 'Come on, Batman!' When they recognised me a few seconds later, they gamely added, 'And Robin!'

Visiting The Oxfordshire Museum in Woodstock, I spied a fantastic building with an expanse of curved windows at the bottom of the garden. It was newly built and still empty; a sign said it was to be the future home of the Soldiers of Oxfordshire Museum, including the regimental museum and archive. Below was another notice asking for volunteers. I had visited a regimental museum before, when researching the war memorial in Barford, and was impressed with their collection of militaria, especially Napoleon's dinner service captured at Waterloo and a WW1 German Maxim machine gun. I was glad it was moving; the museum couldn't reach its potential while it was cluttered and not in a central location. So, drawn in by another opportunity to learn about the impact of war on the lives of people in Oxfordshire, I volunteered at the Soldiers of Oxfordshire Museum in Woodstock throughout its critical first year. I started off working wherever I was needed. Often front of house, where I found chatting with visitors very interesting. Gradually I spent more time with the educational side of the museum, going in at weekends or school holidays to help with the activities.

Occasionally, we would meet a trustee – usually retired White men with a military background. As they were ex-military, they understood the importance of the work of 'other ranks.' They were always keen to meet the volunteers, with that very soldierly directness. One was retired Lieutenant Colonel Ingram Murray, a sprightly, white-haired gentleman. He said, 'You must know my son.' Crossly, I thought his son must be in his fifties and had probably been to public school – there was no chance I knew him. I shook my head. Keeping his patience and managing a determination reserved for the slow and stupid, he tried again, 'Oh, you must ... Alan, Al, the comedian.' I stared blankly as the penny dropped. I was unable to believe that comedian Al Murray, the pub landlord, could have come from such a background. I didn't get to meet him. Another person I didn't get to meet was The Princess Royal at the museum's official opening in September 2014. The building was full of people and she was running a little late as I watched her bustle past my position at the front desk with her entourage of security guards.

Nanny died in April 2013. At her wake, her younger sister, an Irish relative I hadn't met before, spoke with great reverence about their father, William Walsh. Just a collection of apocryphal anecdotes really: 'He was at Gallipoli, then Salonika and then the Middle East' and 'He saved his wounded cousin's life by going out under fire into no man's land to bring him back.' I had been researching my own family, hoping to discover a relative who never came back from the Great War. I desperately wanted someone, somehow, to connect me with the grief and loss felt by so many – similar to the loss I felt myself. I learned of one ancestor who had been a councillor when Stoke-on-Trent was formed, and another who was badly wounded on the Western Front, but was not aware of anything on the Irish side of my family.

Those stories stirred my interest. I knew William had served with the Royal Dublin Fusiliers. With quite a common name and the sketchiness of Irish records, I knew it would not be enough to go on. I had been to Dublin for a weekend with Helen in the mid-90s, following her study of the Irish revolution for A levels, and visited the lonely courtyard where the

1916 rebels were executed in Dublin Castle. I had put my fingers in the bullet holes in the columns outside the post office in Grafton Street. I felt the emotion of those places, and a general connection with the city of Dublin. I studied Irish History myself when I was at university and learned a lot more about the politics, leaders, and the real conflict between fighting for the empire and fighting for your freedom.

In 2014, I wrote a fictional diary entry of an idealised William Walsh at Gallipoli for my creative writing course. I read about the slaughter and bravery of the Irish and other troops on the first day of the disastrous Gallipoli Campaign. The diary entries tried to capture a growing sense of tension as the fictional William made the sea crossing to Gallipoli. I know that idolising people is dangerous; that people are much more complex and nuanced than the family stories that we tell about them. This piece of life writing ended up with William's family in Ireland, who, much to my pride, thought it was from his actual diary and asked to see the rest. I explained that the events were fictional and the setting and other characters were based in fact and thorough research. His grandson shared what he knew about William. This included photos of his Great War medals, with his service number around the side.

I knew from my previous work on First World War soldiers that their service number was a vital piece of information. At last, this was someone I could connect with from this terribly sad period; someone who was brave, someone who did what he believed, had lost everything, and had to put his life back together. I began with his medal records and started to reveal a fascinating man who seemed to have never been to Gallipoli but had spent the war in France and Flanders. He joined up underage and arrived in France in early 1915, just in time to witness the early chlorine gas attacks in the second Battle of Ypres. Their position overrun by the Germans, only 3% of his battalion of 667 survived unwounded. He spent the rest of the war in France and Flanders, survived some of the bloodiest battles and returned to fight over the same ground two years later. He returned home to Dublin by late 1920.

But his story doesn't end there. In 1923, with Ireland tearing itself apart, William took up arms again and joined the Irish Free State army. He transferred to the military police before being discharged for work. When WW2 came, although over 40 and married with seven children, he served with the RAF as an air controller. His speciality was talking down Polish pilots. It has been suggested that Willie, as he liked to be called, didn't speak Polish. Relatives think that his Irish brogue and working knowledge of other languages helped him in this role. William died of throat cancer aged 56 in St Kevin's Hospital, Dublin, in 1953. Had the use of chemical weapons on the Western Front damaged his throat and killed him slowly over his remaining years?

My dad was also unaware of much of the story of

his grandfather and regretted this fact when he first met his future father-in-law, who asked him: 'What did your father do in the war?' Now we knew exactly where he was buried, my dad visited William's grave in the sprawling Glasnevin Cemetery in Dublin and left some flowers. It was probably the first ever visit from someone on our side of the family. A few years later, on our way to Dublin to get the ferry home after a visit to my parents, we visited the village of Dunlavin, County Wicklow, where William grew up with his grandparents. We travelled through the breathtaking rolling hills of the Wicklow Gap, over the winding lanes and views he would have known well.

Settling in to our new home, we decided to try for another baby and were soon pregnant again! The second pregnancy was hard on Helen. Although she had experienced it all before, it wasn't any easier. In the early stages of pregnancy, Helen was very sick. As I was struggling with our new life, Helen suggested we begin a course of counselling. Over the eight-week course, we were surprised at how little and how badly we communicated. We had both constructed unrealistic and unfair versions of each other that we didn't particularly like. Over time, we had accepted these imposters as our real partners and the struggle to live with them was making us unhappy. I think that this 'imposter syndrome' is a common problem in relationships. The answer was to make regular time for each other and to have open, honest communication.

Once again, I was apprehensive about the twenty-week scan, but everything was fine. It told us the gender of the baby: a boy. We had a shortlist of names. I really wanted to name him William after his great-great-grandfather. Although we settled on Bella's name months before the birth, Helen said she would not settle on a name until she had met the baby. The birthing plan was similar to Bella's, except we really wanted to use the birthing pool this time and Helen had once again bravely requested no drugs.

Criss-Cross

I still only knew a handful of people in the village. Our elderly neighbour passed away and, a few months later, we had Sikh neighbours again! Helen was making friends at the school gates and on her dog walks with Tara, and we'd go to the Sports and Social Club with lots of other parents on Friday evenings. When the opportunity to be a parent-governor at the village primary school came up, I applied. I would be using skills and experience I already had: chairing meetings, project work, compliance, and financial oversight. The school had 125 pupils, a new head and had recently been in special measures. There was a lot of work to do. Over the four years I volunteered there, I got to know the staff, other governors and all the parents and pupils. As well as meetings, there were talent shows, assemblies, theatre trips and sports days. I led a school assembly on diversity, led class talks on disability, and workshops on creative writing. Most importantly, it brought me into the community where I had some particularly rewarding experiences.

The first crossover in my volunteering world was when I arranged for the Soldiers of Oxfordshire Museum to hold workshops with every class at Middle Barton Primary School to mark the centenary of the beginning of the First World War. Selected pupils dressed up in replica uniforms as we shared the stories of some of the items from the museum's object handling collection. I enjoyed this form of storytelling, where you could feel the weight and the coldness of an object in your hand and imagine its story.

The museum's object handling collection consisted of a mess tin, an entrenching tool, sewing kit, and a cut-throat razor, which evoked mundane life in the trenches. As many of the men who found themselves in France after 1916 were mostly conscripts, many were skilled craftsmen who would endure long periods of waiting between brief and lethal flurries of activity by making 'trench art' from the plentiful discarded items, such as brass shell cases. The collection included a beautiful tankard with a lid. These moments of activity were represented by a steel helmet, a gas hood, a field dressing, a trench whistle, and a deactivated Mills bomb. 'This wasn't designed to kill; it was designed to hurt as many people as possible,' I would tell the children as they reverently passed it around. The home front was represented by a Queen Mary Christmas gift tin and some home-made knitted socks. A Victory Medal and a death penny covered the aftermath. To make the session more exciting, I took in a deactivated WW1 rifle of my own. The boys especially would marvel at the rifle's sheer weight. I would ask them to imagine carrying it all day or being expected to aim, fire, and reload it at least every three seconds for what was known as the 'mad minute', hitting the target 270m away with at least 15 shots. For this, a marksman received an extra 6p a day. I would use my knowledge of the First World War to deliver object handling workshops and talks on life in the trenches to visiting children from schools all over Oxfordshire. It felt good to be passing on my enthusiasm for this period in history. When I left, I donated my rifle to the museum. It was a better example than the one they had on display.

The next crossover came later that year. I had joined the Parent Teacher Association and saw that it would be enhanced by becoming a charity. It could apply for funding and increase its income by applying for funding from trusts and foundations and claiming gift aid. All these things I had learned in my experience from Ataxia UK. I set up Friends of Middle Barton School (FOMBS) as a charity.

The school's governing body decided to investigate whether or not to become an academy in 2015. Whilst disagreeing with academisation in principle, I worked tirelessly to present a balanced view of it to staff, governors and parents, by assessing local academies, organising drop-ins and workshops over eighteen months. Helen is fiercely opposed to Academisation. For her, it is an transfer of a 'public good' to the greedy private sector – and I was letting it happen. In the face of Helen's anger, I found it difficult to keep an open mind. Keen to improve my understanding of academisation, I became a member of Oxfordshire County Council's Education Scrutiny Committee in May 2016. This enabled me to contribute towards debate on general educational issues and provide feedback on the political progress of the academisation agenda locally.

I was keen to meet other people with ataxia and to ensure that Ataxia UK was doing everything it could to meet their needs. To celebrate Ataxia UK's 50th anniversary in 2015, I visited as many branches and support groups in the Midlands as I could over that summer. Using public transport, I visited 5 groups and featured in the charity's magazine. Helen and I attended Ataxia UK's 50th anniversary dinner in Mayfair, our first black-tie event since Helen's college ball in 2001.

Originally intended to showcase the work of Ataxia UK and the range of therapies available, and to give people a greater understanding of their condition through videos from medical professionals, I helped deliver the first 'All About

Ataxia' workshop at our annual conference. Using my recent experience of getting to know our members, I went around the groups trying to help guide their discussions. As I grew in confidence, I started sharing my own stories and taking people through their diagnosis, helping them to become experts in ataxia and take control of their lives. Amongst other things, we talked about support networks: who is, or should be, in ours. We discussed the importance of knowledgeable and supportive families, friends, and medical professionals. Then, I always asked who had a pet. I delighted in how the room lit up as people talked about their beloved pets, and then got choked up as I explained how Tara, my support dog, saved mine and my family's lives. As the message had shifted to empowering newly diagnosed people, and encouraging those people to take control of their lives – especially through volunteering – I was joined in the workshops by some exceptional people who contributed their own stories. I love catching up with former participants who tell me how their lives have improved since they took the course!

As a school governor, I would spend one afternoon a week reading with the pupils. I enjoyed reading with Bella at home and had made story time part of Billy's bedtime. Knowing how well people reacted to Tara, and as she was insured and trained as a support dog, Mrs Smith, the special educational needs coordinator, agreed to begin using Tara as a reading dog. Helen designed a logo and I had a stamp made so I could stamp the pupils' reading diaries. Helen also drew the logo on a high-vis dog jacket. Tara always knew that when she was wearing that jacket, she was 'working.' I would tell the kids: 'You're reading to Tara, not me. She won't hurry, correct, or judge you.' The trick was to give each child a dog treat, which Tara would sit and wait patiently for. It made a lovely picture. It looked as if Tara was intelligently listening, when in reality she was focused solely on the treat. Soon, I could see the children start to relax and really enjoy reading stories they had brought from home that they thought Tara would like. Anything with picnics or cats in it!

Skydiver

I believed that people with ataxia had to be involved in their charity, run it and raise funds for it. To understand our charity and members better, I trained to take calls on our helpline and administrate our Facebook group for parents with ataxia. Wishing to lead by example, I fundraised via a tandem skydive in 2014. I was surprised at the reaction that followed my decision to jump. Some openly disapproved. They thought I was taking an unnecessary risk. I'm sure it came from a good place, but it still felt like they were saying: 'You're disabled, you shouldn't be doing this.' It just made me want to prove them wrong. Disabled people have to find their own limits. By all means, advise us against taking dangerous and unnecessary risks, but don't try to protect us from living life. Many were supportive. Surprisingly, my GP signed off my medical form after asking a few question, and said: 'You'll really enjoy it' and 'It is one of the safest things that there is to do.' I checked. According to the data provided by British Skydiving (British Skydiving, 2023), the all-time tandem fatality rate since 1990 is about 1 in 930,000 jumps. The World Health Organisation puts a skydive at roughly 46 times safer than travelling by car in the UK. It gets safer when you do a tandem jump with an experienced instructor.

The weather was too poor the first day at the airfield. To give a heavily pregnant Helen a break from her crazy husband, Susan, my mother-in-law, kindly took me on the second day. Finally, the heavy clouds scattered apart and the jumps started. I zipped a jumpsuit over my clothes and was lifted onto the twin propeller plane, my wheelchair staying on the ground. I shuffled backwards and looked out of the window. The plane lurched slightly as it took off. Immediately, the features on the ground looked like a satellite image on Google Maps, slowly losing detail as it is pinched into infinity. The cheerful banter stopped. The smiles had fled. The other jumpers checked their kit and stared straight ahead as we began our climb.

Unfortunately for me, there was time to think. The doubts came. I wondered if I should even be there, given I had a 5-year-old daughter and a son due in a few weeks. Death breathed down the back of my neck. I wondered if he/she had followed me up here, or was he/she waiting for me on the ground with my wheelchair and my distraught mother-in-law? I thought about Neville, my wife's grandfather, who jumped from a burning Halifax bomber in the dark over occupied Holland. I knew something of the fear he must have felt and I silently asked him to watch out for me. For the first time ever, my future was wide open. I didn't know what was going to happen to me. And I didn't like it.

Then we're sitting on the edge of the door, my feet dangle into the emptiness. Above the clouds, the sky is a solid azure and the air feels saturated with ice. The memory of the walk-in freezer at the fast-food restaurant I worked in as a teenager flashes through my mind. The air rushes past. I can't see my instructor; he is behind me. I shut my eyes. Time slows down. I think: 'Please go, please go,' over and over again like a mantra. Finally, we tumble out into the freezing sunlight. My stomach turns as we instantly accelerate to 120mph. I want to go limp, to shut down, to hide, to let this whole ordeal wash over me. The wind thunders in my ears as we fall.

My instructor taps me on the shoulder; the cameraman is right in front of me. Far from happy, I remember to smile. I am trying to stay alive, trying to figure out which way up I am, where the ground is and to remember to keep breathing. We begin to spin. I close my eyes and brace myself. We go faster and faster. I taste sick and can't take much more. I am just about to beg the instructor to stop when our spin is cut short. The cameraman is in front of us again. Once more I look up and try to smile as the air pushes all the muscles on my face into a tortured grimace.

The chute opens and we are pulled roughly upward into the clouds. The jolt as we change speed is not as bad as I expect. We are enveloped by an eerie silence. I release the breath I realise have been holding in. My thoughts are broken as I see an object flash past us in the corner of my eye.

I think my shoe has come off. 'I'm never going to get that back.' I smile as I imagine my shoe appearing out of the sky and mystifying any nearby people, or animals, as it thuds to the ground. I try to say that my shoe has gone; the instructor assures me that the falling object I saw shooting past was just the cameraman. I look down. With relief, I see that my shoes are still with me. We break through the clouds; the fields below lie in a peaceful patchwork of summer shades. I realise I *have* left everything down on the ground, other people, disability, responsibility, shame, my wheelchair. For the first time ever, I am just me Finally, my mind is clear ... lost in that beautiful moment.

'Can you put your feet on mine?' the instructor asks, as we had agreed earlier. I can just reach the tops of my knees with my hands. I grab the material of my jumpsuit and pull. The muscles in my legs have tensed and I can't bend them. I cannot touch his feet with mine. I cannot even get near them. He is five foot five at best; I am six. I relax. 'We'll try again,' he says with an edge of frustration. I try again, nothing. The danger becomes real when the instructor shouts, 'This is very important; we'll both be very badly hurt if we can't get your legs up.' Rather than motivating me, this terrifies me. I grab the material of the jumpsuit and pull with everything I have, screaming with the effort. The muscles in my legs are on fire, my knees still locked. I have pulled the legs of my jumpsuit over my knees. We are quite low now. We are out of time. 'This is not good; if you can lift your legs at all, do it now!' the instructor orders. I lift, but there was nothing left. How fitting, I thought, my body has let me down once again, one last spectacular time. I never wanted to hurt anyone else, I'm not ready to die. We come in fast, people shouting and scurrying over the grassy landing area. I close my eyes and brace myself for the pain, like in a nightmare. I accept that I won't be opening them again.

There is a thud. My bare knees hit the ground; there is a sharp pain there. I am winded as both our bodies hit the ground, mine beneath. My face hits the ground hard. My instructor quickly releases his harness and climbs off me. I hear voices, urgent, worried. I am rolled over, people stand over me, the sun flashing between them so I can't see their faces. I still have no breath. The pain in my knees eases. I can't be paralysed, or dead. My legs are both there, my exposed knees grazed and one side of my face sore. I'm elated because I have survived, and just as exhausted. Someone keeps asking if I am OK. I'm still winded, only able to answer with a grunt. I don't know myself yet. The cameraman returns to capture the after-jump reaction. 'How was it?' he asks. 'Great' I say, shakily sticking a thumb up and smiling.

I'm really glad that I had such an amazing experience and raised money for Ataxia UK. I would highly recommend a tandem skydive to anyone. I'm sure that with better preparation, I would have enjoyed it even more. I don't think there was any real danger; my instructor used all his skill and experience to bring us in at a shallow angle. Nevertheless, Helen made me promise there would be no more crazy fundraising stunts. I have no desire to do it again myself anyway! Afterwards was just as interesting. Those people who had such low expectations of me were now saying that I was very brave. I thought a lot about this. Was I brave? Were they saying: 'You're brave because you are disabled and did something physically difficult?' I never felt brave; I was terrified and wanted it to stop. People were using their idea of disability to process what I'd done. I didn't care as long as they paid up! I never once thought I was being courageous like the superheroes I admired as a child. I spent most of my brief time in the sky feeling incredibly anxious or uncomfortable and the remainder thinking silly or mundane thoughts. I was only in awe of the silent beauty I drifted through for a few seconds. Bella, just 5 at the time, thought the hat

I wore to jump out of the plane was silly. For me, that was the best response of all.

With my parents now living in Ireland, Helen's were on standby to drive to the maternity centre in Chipping Norton. Helen felt confident that she would be able to drive us both there. That's *real* bravery for you. Our experienced midwife extended her shift to make sure the birth went well. She came out to our home several times to check on Helen's progress and eventually to induce labour. I tried to help too. Once again, I had made a CD and tried to make sure we had everything we would need. This time, she made it to the birthing pool and the seemed to be easier for her. The baby was pressed into her arms in the dimly lit room. Helen looked into his eyes and said: 'Hello, Billy!' It was strange going back to the world of nappies, crying, and bottle feeding. Bella was in her own bed at 5 years old and had just started school, – we knew there was light at the end of the tunnel!

On days out I doubled once again as a pram, and the sling that I had used to secure Bella to my chest made a return. Helen also had a more substantial baby carrier that was like a rucksack, which left her hands-free to hold Tara's lead, Bella's hand, or push me along. Not for the first time, I greatly admired her strength and fortitude.

I was pleased with the direction that Ataxia UK was taking. United by the ambition of encouraging steady growth and increasing professionalism, the board created and invested in a Fundraising Team, helped develop a world-class Research Team, improved the processes of our Finance Team, built a digital presence, and brought in much-needed administrative support for our chief exec. As we built this foundation, we completed some exciting projects and campaigns. We introduced a striking new logo, moved to a new office, and ran the Fractured Lives campaign. I took a special interest in projects that put people with ataxia at the very centre of our charity. We developed the 16–30 group to hear the voices of young people with ataxia, sought to add an element of challenge, and through our conferences championed the many achievements of people with ataxia, and we targeted bringing volunteers in through the InControl project. I cannot take credit for any of these, but I influenced them. Through it all has been our CEO, Sue Millman. A selfless, incredible person who works as hard as three people.

Emancip8 access consultancy

Even though I was busier and happier than I'd ever been, I still felt the pull of capitalism in the shape of earning money from my knowledge and expertise. Soon after moving to Middle Barton, I started my own access consultancy. As a member of the National Register of Access Consultants, I anticipated that Emancip8 would offer specialised advice on access issues and training in disability awareness to employers throughout Oxfordshire and the UK. Helen would be my assistant. I attended specialist training in London and bought the tools, books and memberships required. To qualify, I conducted audits in my own time for Middle Barton Sports and Social Club, Wantage Leisure Centre, and the Mill Arts Centre in nearby Banbury. I also gave free access advice for the George Inn, Barford St Michael, Middle Barton School, Middle Barton Stores, and Ataxia UK. I even had business cards printed and designed a website.

I had a bad cold before the final interview and took a chance on going to London. The panel asked me to begin my presentation when I was ready. Embarrassed, I explained that I had been ill recently and had missed this detail and hadn't prepared anything, but would speak to any questions they asked. It was awkward. I thought I had made the best of it. When I received feedback on the audits I had submitted for interview, they had found issues with those too. I was also disappointed that all three of the panel were middle-class White men, each with no visible disability, and a little offended that they could question my judgement. I was invited to reapply in the future. As it would have to be a new application, I felt I had missed my chance. Resubmitting would mean completing another batch of audits for free, doing the costly training again and renewing my expensive insurance and memberships. I had lots of other things happening, so I let it go.

On the Buses

Aware of my interaction with local politicians about the proposed cuts to public transport in my village, due to a letter published in the local paper, Steeple Barton Parish Council asked me to join the Oxfordshire County Council's Parish Transport group to keep the parish informed about the proposed cuts. I travelled by bus from our village to the meeting in Oxford. The bus was almost empty and ran far too frequently. Having worked in local government and understanding how austerity works, I instinctively knew the group was being prepared for bad news. Classic divide-and-rule tactics. Each delegate was only there to defend their own narrow interests; the proposed cuts were phased so as to minimise objection. Nobody was looking at the bigger picture.

Back in Middle Barton, we had a public meeting. I gave my report and dramatically declared, 'The writing is on the wall, we need to have a Plan B.' Some wonderful people with skills and experience stepped forward to help. As an experienced trustee, I took on the task of leading the group and registering it as a charity and a company in August 2016, and organised and chaired those early committee meetings, helping to start a company, put together a business plan, open a bank account and apply for the start-up funding we desperately needed. Today, OurBus Bartons provides affordable, daily, timetabled transport for members of the public residing in or visiting The Bartons and surrounding villages in West Oxfordshire. We operate nine routes, serving eleven destinations and cover over 2,000 miles a month. We cover running costs with fares and small donations. Large donations or grants are needed to cover capital costs. OurBus Bartons links local villages with rail and bus transport hubs and nearby towns. There are also daily early and evening runs to connect with rail and main bus services for both commuters and students travelling from local villages to Banbury, Oxford, or London.

I coordinated safety training for our new volunteer drivers, developed a website, social media accounts, created a 'hire procedure' and 'accessible journey' statement, and built links with local media. In a nod to my previous experience of running charities, the agenda for our first management committee meeting was neatly divided into financial, operational, driver, fundraising and passengers, with reports for each being shared in advance, so each committee member could update the others. Special mention to my fellow directors, and especially Martin, the beating heart of OurBus Bartons. He drove all the routes himself, registered them and produced our timetables. Using his contacts in the transport industry, he found us our first bus and keeps our current ones running. Just six months after the devastating and total loss of public transport in our community, we had founded OurBus Bartons Ltd, a volunteer-led charitable company providing transport solutions to people within our community.

Crowdfunding

By this point, I had successfully raised funds for Ataxia UK, OurBus Bartons and Middle Barton School. It was time to use this expertise to improve my own life. I needed a reliable and more powerful means of getting around. At home, I was OK. I had to rely on others to do anything outside the house. Just moving around in my wheelchair was becoming more of a struggle. Often, observers would ask, 'Why don't you get an electric chair?' I'm not sure how that grim instrument of capital punishment would help my situation. I think they meant a powerchair! What a great idea; I wish I had thought of that! However, I gave a very practical reply, 'I want to maintain the little physical activity I have; it wouldn't actually fit into most London taxis and buses; and it would certainly be too heavy for my wife to lift into our car.' They nodded with sympathy, but I know that my convenient excuses were just that. I was avoiding facing up to my worsening mobility.

After a lot of encouragement and careful consideration, I arranged to try out a trike attachment made by a Spanish company called BATEC, which make a variety of handcycles. These clamp onto any manual wheelchair and turn it into a speedy electric trike. This option meant I could use it to travel a good distance, then disconnect it and enter buildings in my own wheelchair. Their website declares: 'You can get used to being in a wheelchair, but not to giving up on life!' That was reassuring! With its chunky tyre, disc brakes and headlight, it really is a good-looking piece of engineering that turns heads. I recorded a video of me zooming along my street during my trial and put it on Facebook for fun. When a friend commented, 'You need this in your life!' that got me thinking.

Without the new carbon-fibre wheelchair the rep recommended, the electric front wheel attachment itself cost £5000, which I knew I could not afford. Knowing that disabled people are mostly on their own when it comes to covering the extra costs of being disabled, and that trusts and charities might be able to help, I decided to crowdfund the £5000 myself. Crowdfunding involves appealing to a large number of people to each give a portion of money. If your crowd is big enough, you can raise some significant funds. This idea is big in America. In the UK, your crowd is usually much smaller but give much more. I don't consider asking for the support of others as begging if your appeal carries a super positive message and nothing to inspire sympathy or pity. My campaign for 'life-changing mobility equipment' began. The generosity of friends and family, a community event, and some funding from Barchester Charity got me over the line.

When I thanked everyone who had supported my appeal, I said the trike would change my life and it has in so many ways. Doing things on my own has greatly improved my confidence, especially on holidays and family days out. I've travelled by train to football matches at Wembley Stadium, taken a full part in village life, explored a French fishing village and several National Trust nature reserves. Things I never thought I'd do. I found myself on my own again for the first time in years. Once I got used to this scary new feeling, I began to rediscover the simple pleasure of being alone.

My trike has helped me as a dad too. Instead of holding everyone back on days out to the grounds of stately homes, parks, or weekend city breaks and holidays, I can scout ahead and give thrilling rides to our youngest when he gets tired. I have taken charge of my two kids on a cycle ride at Center Parcs (ideal for trikes!), my daughter for a pub lunch in a neighbouring village and would often be with the other parents on the playground of the village school at home time.

According to SCOPE, a disability charity in England and Wales, we live in a society where two thirds of us are uncomfortable talking to a disabled person. In the same way a support dog helps re-establish the link between disabled people and others, I have found that people smile and wave when they see me whizzing through the village, zipping around Cork Market, navigating the medieval cobbled town of Carcassonne, on a daring solo mission around Swansea Bay, along a windswept Norfolk coastal path or across London on a summer night. The way people think about disabled people has been challenged by the presence of my trike because it makes me more approachable. Lots of people ask me about it. My trike is a very elegant solution to my worsening mobility; it has given me hundreds of miles and many moments of happiness. It's a great privilege to have it. When people ask how I got it, I answer that it was a precious gift from my friends, family, and my community. It really has changed my life.

Having survived its first eighteen months and still the only operation of its kind, OurBus Bartons found itself at the forefront of a national debate. We received a visit from the Under Secretary of State for Transport Jesse Norman MP in January 2018 and were represented on the All-Party Parliamentary Group for Community Transport. We featured in the Community Transport Association's magazine in Spring 2018 and responded to the Department for Transport's White Paper on the future of community transport. I also appeared on local radio and two BBC South Politics' General Election TV specials to champion the importance of transport for the community.

By juggling being a Trustee of Ataxia UK and a school governor, I had learned a lot about myself, teamwork, leadership, and disability. A big personal lesson came when I took my re-election in 2016 for granted, did little to prepare and lost. I learned that to represent others properly, you must do the work. Rather than lose me, my fellow trustees decided to co-opt me to the board so I could stand in the next election (which I won!). This really boosted my confidence. I was voted in as vice chair the following year.

2016 was a very low point for me. After a few seasons circling the drain, Aston Villa were finally relegated from the Premier League. We also had what I think was a fraudulent Brexit referendum and Donald Trump. On top of all that, we lost David Bowie, Gene Wilder, Carrie Fisher, and George Michael. During the Brexit referendum, I told people it was a terrible idea: freedom of movement, human rights, and food standards would go. It was clearly to allow the super-rich to continue avoiding paying taxes. I was bitterly disappointed my mum allowed herself to be swept along with the lies and voted to leave anyway, telling me she had done it to ensure a better life for my kids.

In February 2017, I successfully applied for funding to support FOMBS' first major project: the conversion of an unused outdoor pool area into an outdoor classroom or eco area. The final design was based on the ideas of the pupils. Work began in the summer of 2017. However, that winter we realised that the contractor had gone into liquidation and that the first phase of work was of a low standard. With legal support from Helen's mum, we tried to recover our investment.

I contributed to the school's OFSTED inspection that May. As chair of the school's Standards and

Performance Committee, I ensured consistent coverage of the curriculum and that all policies and functions fully supported the school's progress in the months leading up to it. The school maintained its 'good' rating. The positive impact of the school's reading dog was proudly mentioned in the OFSTED inspection report.

One evening that summer, my uncle and I were discussing how the honours system recognises too many politicians and business leaders and not enough people who really benefit their own communities. The next day, I decided that I would have to buy a ticket and make a good thing happen – I asked him to test our assumption by nominating me. After all, if you have a vague hope that something good might happen, it probably won't. Because I had initiated the process, I obviously had no ethical issues with accepting an honour if I was offered one. For me, it is simply recognition of one's good work, and it could be used to help people. I provided contact details for people I knew who I thought could help. Our MP, Robert Courts, who had been at the first Ourbus Bartons public meeting, was a key supporter. Once a detailed application had been submitted, my uncle received a polite acknowledgement that his nomination had been received and advised that if he did not hear anything in two years, he could assume it had been unsuccessful. He cleverly made sure that the application remained current by submitting updates over the next two years. Helen kindly called this work: 'Project Satan'. I told a few close friends about the nomination and swore them to secrecy; partly because I felt embarrassed telling people about something that would probably not happen.

My last meeting as a governor ended dramatically. We were to make the final decision on whether or not to become an academy. I had learned that as charities themselves, academies were not all chasing profit for their shareholders and that bigger chains were able to deliver efficiency savings amongst their operations. There were benefits, but it was very important to join the right one. However, convinced that education should continue to be a Universal Basic Service (Anna Coote, 2020), I still argued that we should not become an academy as a matter of principle; education is not a commodity, but a social good and should be managed by the state and the community. Allowing the private sector to get involved would lead to rising costs and falling standards. All the other governors voted to make the school an academy over the coming summer. I saw little value in being an academy governor, so when my term expired I did not restand. Considering the pressure I had felt from Helen, it was a relief to finally put the whole episode behind me. Five years later, I think we chose the best academy chain possible, and Billy's experience there is not too different from when Bella attended as a state school pupil. It is important for volunteers to constantly seek new challenges and not get taken for granted, and I already knew what I wanted to do. The most enjoyable aspect of my time as a school governor was me and Tara the Reading Dog interacting with the pupils. I really enjoyed getting to know the children and seeing them grow in confidence.

Tara passed away at our home in December 2018 after a year of battling cancer. Saying goodbye was so very hard. At the end we did the best thing for her, not us. We buried her in our back garden with all the love she deserved. From helping Helen face her depression and preparing to be a mum, to helping me adjust to retirement, making me feel a part of the world around us again, guarding us like we were royalty, and giving us her companionship and unconditional love, Tara made us better people and saved us all. She even saved Christmas once! When Bella was very young, I told her that a very agitated Santa had knocked on our door on Christmas Eve and explained that he had landed his team of reindeers on our roof and Rudolph, who was his navigator, needed a rest. He had heard that we had a very special dog and asked if he could borrow her to guide him round the village. I agreed, and Tara saved Christmas for everyone in our village.

We found her absence to be so painful. A hurt that did not lessen as time went on. As Christmas came with its messages of renewal and hope, we realised we didn't have to replace Tara to move on. We welcomed Treacle, our new Airedoodle puppy, a month later.

In March 2019, I was invited to become a director of Mobility Matters Campaign Ltd, the national representative of Community Transport Operators, which provided evidence in a landmark judicial review brought against The Department of Transport by big commercial operators jealously guarding their profits and seeking to push community transport operators away from taking paid work. Even though OurBus Bartons doesn't tender for contract work, the outcome of this review would determine the future sustainability of the entire community transport sector. I represented small and voluntary providers through this important process.

That May, we began an innovative arrangement with Middle Barton School to use our third bus during term time to collect children for the school's breakfast club. The school provided a driver and we refuelled and maintained the bus. Everybody won. The school had access to cheap and safe transport, parents knew their children were arriving at school safely, and we had a spare bus if needed.

LIVING WITH DYING

Two big losses in my family in 2019 reminded me how close we all are to death. My cousin spencer died suddenly at the age of 41 in July 2019 and my nephew, Hayden, died in October, aged just 20.

We are surrounded by death. Death is an important part of life, but disabled people know only too well that death is only one trauma away. For me, a big part of having an incurable and progressive condition is accepting you will have a shorter life as a result. When you know life is short and that anything can happen, you have to live in the moment. It is a truth that other people glimpse, yet can't seem to hold on to. I have had a chance to stop and look around. With my condition, I know I have no choice but to live in the present and try to be grateful for what I can.

What shapes our understanding of death? Ourselves and our traditions and rituals. In his 2020 book, *No Time like the Present* (Fox, 2020), Michael J. Fox talks about the passing of his father-in-law as a positive experience. 'A letting go, unforced and natural [...] the prevailing mood and spirit around Stephen, gratitude, was the very essence of the man.' His father-in-law had carefully prepared his friends and family to accept his death by the way he lived his life. It is for those who are left behind to deal with death, so it should not be a taboo subject. Rather, it should be discussed openly and often and all the necessary arrangements made.

Despite my acceptance of death, I find funerals difficult because they are purposefully laden with moments that trigger extreme emotional responses and are a concentrated and dramatic copy of this journey through loss to acceptance. All in 90 minutes! We are brought as close to death as possible with the arrival of the coffin, only to welcome the understanding that our lives are short, and our loved ones will live on in our memories and actions. Then we sing a hymn in celebration and go home.

A great example of how this process *should* work is captured in a favourite story of mine: Charles Dickens' *A Christmas Carol*. Scrooge (Dickens, 2022) comes to a revelation after he views his own grave. He is changed forever and finds redemption in bringing joy to others and living in the moment. He can't just forget what he has learned and move on.

Death is a recurring character in my life. I first met him in Terry Pratchett's excellent Discworld books; me a young teenager and him a giant skeleton, wrapped in a cowl and carrying a scythe. His booming monosyllabic voice always emphasised IN CAPITALS. He spoke with the clarity and wisdom of a timeless observer. I find he often recurs in my own writing. We met again in Neil Gaiman's *Sandman* (Gaiman, 2020). This time in the guise of an ageless, precocious teenage girl, just trying to help people move on – whether they are ready or not. I like the way both of these characters are benign caretakers, somehow kind and gentle – like old friends. This is the death who comes for everyone; it is better to accept the visit and not be afraid.

Beginning with my diagnosis of Friedreich's ataxia, I felt closer to death. I had to confront my own mortality again when Helen and I chose to become parents in 2008 with Bella, and again in 2013 with Billy. Another unwelcome reminder occurred in 2011, when I took medical retirement. Such was the seriousness of the medical retirement process that, by the end of it, I was convinced that I had a few months left to live. Co-signing a thirty-year mortgage with my wife in 2013 reminded me, once again, that I would not live to make the final payment at the age of 67. My assessment for Personal Independence Payment has been hanging over me since 2013. There is nothing like an impending state review into your disability to make you continuously and painfully aware of your own mortality. Similarly, I felt as though I had a brush with death during my skydive in 2014.

As with many neurological conditions, each person's progression is different, but I accept that I will reach a point at which I will enter a final decline. I want to be in control and avoid a painful and undignified end. I was alarmed to learn that the current law does not work for dying people. In England, Wales and Northern Ireland, assisting a suicide is a crime. Those convicted could face up to fourteen years in prison. Most importantly, it is unlawful for medical professionals here to assist.

Dying people (with six months or less to live) rightly deserve support to bring a peaceful end to their lives at home. In a poll of 5000 people in 2019, 84% of the British public supported the legalisation of assisted dying and, according to a 2015 poll, so do 86% of disabled people. Despite this support, in September 2021, the British Medical Association made the decision to adopt a neutral position on assisted dying. Of course, if the process of assisted dying must become heavily medicalised, we need to trust medical professionals. Some disabled people argue that safeguards in the UK Bill would limit the powers of the act to very few in immense pain at the ends of their lives. Others argue that if it becomes law, these safeguards would be watered down by those in power, making assisted suicide an easy option for distressed disabled people, especially those with intellectual disabilities and their families. While I understand the complexities of preventing the abuse of an assisted death service, forcing people to travel abroad and pay thousands of pounds for a dignified death is cruel and wrong.

More importantly, can we trust a government that was found by the High Court not to have consulted with disabled people on its recent National Disability Strategy? And that has been condemned twice in recent years by the UN for its treatment of disabled people?

Death comes to all of us. It brings grief. There's no sweeping it under the rug. It makes me wonder why, after it touching our lives, don't we all live our lives with direction, clarity and gratitude by bringing joy to others? Why doesn't everyone who has been touched by grief go forwards with a new understanding of the shortness of life and the importance of living in the moment? I think that death is best to answer this: 'MORTAL LIFE JUST DOESN'T LET YOU STOP FOR LONG ENOUGH TO LOOK AROUND. AND WHEN YOU DO, IT'S TOO LATE.'

My cousin, Spencer

His loss changed my life. My maternal aunt and her family had always been very kind and generous to me. As a surly teenager, they took me on a family holiday to Florida with them. Perhaps his parents' example helped form a young Spencer's ideas of generosity that he would carry with him for the rest of his life. His father nominated me for my MBE; although Spencer was aware of that, the actual award was made after he died. As someone who celebrated all things British, I think he would have been especially proud of his cousin.

Spencer and his older brother, Grant, both attended public schools, boarding at the prestigious Westminster School in London from the age of 11. I can only imagine what that must have been like, how that felt. I do know that when we are tested, strong bonds are forged with those we share that experience with. As well as the high standard of education, pupils have access to life-changing networks and opportunities. Spencer seized those opportunities and worked hard to become the very best. He was a master scuba diver, an authority on marine architecture, and a world champion debater. He chaired Oxford Union's debating society whilst at university.

We had spent time together as children, but rarely saw each other as adults. Our busy lives had moved us away from that happy childhood bubble. I would hear bits of his news through our mums, so I had an idea that Spencer was an especially generous and kind person. He was a beloved godfather to many children all around the world and had a strong network of friends who held him in the very highest regard. He always remembered my family's birthdays and came to my surprise 40th birthday party. It was a surprise to me I had lasted that long! He was one of the few people I felt compelled to give a big hug to whenever I saw him. On one of those rare occasions,

I must have mentioned that sitting in our new garden was problematic because of the strong sun in the afternoons. A few days later, I received a text from Spencer warning me to expect a call from a local garden centre to arrange delivery of a cantilever parasol. He had also paid for installation. I was to learn that this fixing of many problems in such a grand style was a typical Spencerian gesture.

After many attempts, we finally had dinner with Spencer. He arrived on time in an electric car laden with gifts: fine wine and chocolates for my wife and I, and birthday presents for both our children. We were fascinated as he told us about diving off the Bahamas onto the remains of the Vulcan bomber that was built for the 1965 Bond film, *Thunderball*. We listened enthralled as he explained how nature had reclaimed the wreck and it was now home to turtles, lobsters and moray eels. Just six weeks later, when our son unwrapped his birthday gift from 'Cousin Spencer', a moment of great sadness overcame us as we explained that Spencer had died just a few weeks earlier.

Through working closely with his friends to honour his memory, I learned what a great man he actually was. It was very apparent at Spencer's funeral that his generosity was habitual and he had become something of a legend. His friends filled the church, coming from all over the world to say goodbye. The eulogies revealed how Spencer had provided a calm, fatherly influence, just when his friends needed it most. He would take a problem and solve it, giving his advice, help, support or, most importantly, his time. Exactly as he had for us, he was always willing to help his friends time and time again. That sort of generosity is never forgotten.

I saw that his friends had set up a memorial page on Facebook paying tribute to him and promising to honour his memory in a lasting way. I reached out and offered my help. One of his friends, on his way to a New Year's Eve party in Upstate New York, called back the next day to welcome me on board. Evidence that Spencer's friends operated in a different world to me! Spencer's headstone declares his name, dates, and a simple three-word epitaph: A Great Man. Now I understand why. Spencer's greatness was evident in how he approached life. He knew that generosity has a ripple effect, touching people far beyond the original recipients for many years. I'm proud to have known him and was excited to continue his legacy. In a small way, I wanted to help his closest friends to work through their grief. His final, unintended and most generous gift to me was for me to get to know them.

A PAST LIFE

I had always wanted to do past-life regression. I was open to the idea of having a past life, but couldn't see how it worked mathematically ... with more people alive today than have lived throughout history, how can we all have a past life? We may have been animals, insects or in one of the parallel universes created each time an individual makes a decision. The possibilities are endless, which explains why there are so many Napoleons. Really, I just wanted to see how creative my mind was at constructing an alternative life. I had always been amazed by the work of hypnotist and illusionist Derren Brown. I decided to 'buy a ticket' and got in touch with a past life regression therapist: Louise.

I got comfortable, relaxed, and we started. I remember being quite aware as Louise counted me down. I felt very relaxed, sort of like approaching the edge of sleep. I had seen stage hypnotists and was expecting to fall into a deep trance. Perhaps to begin clucking like a chicken. Instead, I remember feeling embarrassed and thinking: 'This isn't working; I'll just have to go along with this.' After some more soothing and counting, Louise asked me to think of a special day and asked where I was and what I was doing. I told her it was my son's wedding day, and I was looking for my husband. The service could not happen without him. Louise asked me to describe where I was. 'I'm inside a large tent; it's so hot, but the air is moving as we are near a big river, but oh, the insects.' I liked this detail. Seeing I was settled with an individual, Louise asked: 'What is your name?' 'Kareema,' I replied. Moving on, Louise explained: 'We're leaving this time and moving to your last day, where are you?' I responded straight away, continuing the earlier theme of being disappointed with my husband, 'I am at home, it is dark, my family are here, I am waiting for my husband, someone is stroking my hand, I can hear prayers. I'm so tired, but not afraid.'

Afterwards, I was interested in the details I gave, and congratulated myself on not choosing to construct the obvious past life like Anne Boleyn, Joan of Arc, or the Great War soldier I could have believingly made up. I wasn't convinced there was anything in it. At the very least, it gave me an interesting story to tell. Louise had recorded our session and emailed it to me a few days later. When I played it back, I was quite shocked. I didn't recognise my own voice. At the end, I was breathless, almost whispering, frail. When I said, 'I'm so tired, but not afraid', it was a resolute statement. I really don't remember doing any acting! At the very least, I might have the potential for becoming more adept at meditating. That I had 'chosen' someone obsessed with themselves, appearances, and family didn't strike me as odd until writing this. Perhaps 'Kareema', the overbearing mother, is more of a part of my own personality than I understand.

ARCh reader

The ARCh Oxfordshire (Assisted Reading for Children) award-winning volunteer programme I had seen on Twitter looked ideal. You work twice a week with the same three children over an entire school year. The emphasis is on passing on your love of reading through mentoring, building a relationship and getting to know each other. As the school makes a financial contribution, your efforts are much more valued and appreciated. As an ARCh reader, you are issued with a box full of books and games to really engage the children. You can swap these for others at regular book-swapping events.

Reassuringly, the process of becoming an ARCh volunteer was very stringent. I had an interview to join the scheme. I took our new puppy, Treacle, to the interview, explaining that one day I was hoping she would become their first reading dog. My interviewers agreed and welcomed me to the scheme! I think Tara would be very proud of the positive influence she has had on us all. Next came comprehensive training and several certificates to earn before my supervisor, who I recognised as a previous volunteer driver with OurBus Bartons, arranged for me to work with a primary school in Banbury where John was chair of governors and Helen tutored one day a week. So, at least getting there would not be a problem.

The school had worked with ARCh before, so they already understood our function. I joined another new volunteer for our induction. With a smile, the head teacher told my female colleague, 'We have some lovely early readers for you.' She turned to me and said, 'We have some year five boys that have attendance problems and will really benefit from spending time with you.' My heart sank a little.

Our first session was at the start of term in September and went very well. Although all three boys were visibly nervous, they were able to tell me a bit about themselves. All three said that reading was their favourite hobby – I think they were just saying what they thought I wanted to hear! We began by using a general mixture of books and games and getting to know one another. I was generous with praise and tried to structure our sessions, letting the children determine the kind of activity we did. Often, one of the boys was absent and I would read with other members of the class. They were lovely; I really enjoyed meeting them and hearing a bit of their stories. I guiltily wondered how much nicer it would be for me if I had been working with these children instead. On Thursdays, I would go in with Helen and spend the morning assisting in the classroom before my afternoon session. I got to help the children with their spelling and mathematics. This helped me settle into the class.

With one of my assigned children often absent, and only making slow progress with the other two, my confidence began to falter. In an education system that fails so many children, I wasn't sure if I had the skills or the time to give the help mine needed. I wasn't sure if I was wasting my time and theirs. It wasn't until I attended 'recall' training with the other members of my class who had also started volunteering in schools that I realised that most of us were working with children with challenging behaviours. I also learned that many ARCh volunteers often do not begin to see the benefits of their work until after Christmas.

I stuck with it and had some success. As we were looking through an atlas, one of my boys started telling me about the Titanic. Although his knowledge seemed mostly related to the film, I could see that this subject really captured his imagination, so I bought in a couple of books from home. Over the next couple of weeks, we explored nautical terms, Morse code, shipbuilding, and the facts of the disaster. I even came back after half term with a Titanic quiz, which he did very well at. So, I knew he had been listening after all.

I always introduced myself as Richard and it is lovely to be greeted in that way in the corridors. I think word has spread. Some children from other classes saw me with my children and were interested in reading with me. From listening to them read, you get to join them in their amazing worlds. Sadly, it is also clear that many haven't fully developed their reading skills and don't have any opportunity to interact with grown-ups. My two readers have now both finished their first books with me; I have read with the others in the class and have had my supervision, which went really well. I hadn't missed a session and was enjoying them more each time. A clue to this is that I have been referring to them over the last few paragraphs as 'my' children!

Not for the first time, I saw the links between all the voluntary work I had undertaken and my growing feeling of fulfilment. OurBus Bartons was growing and adapting to fit its community. In February 2019, a local day centre lost its funding for transport. With several members living in Middle Barton, we quickly restructured our services so the members could travel to the day centre using their bus passes. Thanks to donations, our first new bus, named Bella the Bus, arrived in March 2019 and went straight into service. We officially launched the bus at our annual general meeting that June, with Bella and our MP cutting the ribbon.

I was very proud to be made an ambassador for Ataxia UK at their conference in 2018. At the same conference, I also ran a workshop in which I tried to convince delegates that while Brexit was a terrible idea, a chaotic, unmanaged Brexit would have significant consequences for people with disabilities. We had already seen medical research partnerships move away from the UK. I warned that our rights were under attack and warned of a government operating beyond the control of parliament.

The year brought some sadness. My parents broke up. They had not been getting on for a while. My advice to them both was to find happiness separately while they had the time. This proved a lot easier for my dad than for my mum. They both met new partners, yet a lack of money tied them to an uneasy sharing of their home in Ireland until recently.

With our attempt to recover the deposit we had paid to the company that were building our eco area at a dead end, Helen stepped in and rallied local parents with professional expertise to both correct and finish the work that had already been started. This included a new roof. As Helen is a much better completer/finisher than I, the school's outdoor classroom was opened in summer 2019, thanks to her.

Safe roads

The first superhero I ever met was David Prowse (Darth Vader from *Star Wars*). I was disappointed that this giant of a man was not dressed as Darth Vader, he was the Green Cross Code Man. His catchphrase was "Stop, look, listen." That is precious advice on how to cross roads, which I have passed on to my kids.

When a friend was involved in a serious incident while crossing the main road running through our village, I set up the Safe Roads for Middle Barton campaign group. I added an online petition to the written one already in circulation, calling on our elected representatives to 'take urgent and decisive action to address the problem of speeding vehicles through our village.' Like David Prowse, making the world a safer place was more important to me.

The B4030 is a fast and busy road that runs between Bicester and Chipping Norton and serves a busy industrial estate and a large employer. This road runs through Middle Barton (population 1500) as North Street, cutting the village in half. The primary school and preschool are on one side, the majority of homes built in the last sixty years on the other. Many families must cross this busy road twice a day.

Although there have never been any fatalities, speeding traffic has caused lots of injuries and damage to property. It quickly became clear that this was a long-standing and complex issue. After listening to people and reading their impassioned comments on our petition, I realised that everyone had their own perception on the causes of, and solutions to, the problem. But it was always someone else's fault. The mums on the school run, local people, lorry drivers, tractor drivers, or just outsiders. This problem was this very human one. For all of us, the other cars are the traffic jam or the congestion; we think we are the only ones on an important journey. When we grind to a halt in traffic, we become part of the problem without realising.

Back to Scrooge again. He blames other people. By loaning money at barely affordable interest to those who cannot really afford it, he is very much a cause of the poverty he can see all around him. This is definitely how I was supposed to feel about the tenants of Birmingham City Council.

This lack of empathy is also a common difficulty for activism. By their nature, people focus on their little part of the problem and lose the overall aim of the group they are in. They have their own issues and dominate meetings, lobby and agitate to resolve them – and then, their work done, they quietly disappear. Sometimes, it's about who you know and how much money you have. Our community liaison police officer told us about a small traffic calming scheme in a neighbouring village that was completed very quickly because the entire scheme was privately funded by a resident who was married to a former government minister's daughter.

After this petitioning and information gathering stage, we distributed a press release just before Christmas and it was picked up by our local media. For once, I was pleased with the dramatic headline in the *Banbury Guardian*: 'Enough is Enough. Someone Will Get Killed, Say Villagers.' The foreshadowing of tragedy reinforced our frustration. With the profile of our issue raised, I met with local politicians and decision-makers and formally delivered a 352 strong petition to Oxfordshire County Council's cabinet meeting in January 2020.

Oxfordshire County Council's formal response promised significant traffic-calming work would be carried out. Funding was dependant on a large development nearby and no timescale was given. To keep focus on the issue, we called on our supporters to back the 'Community Speedwatch' initiative running in the village. This is a group of locals who deploy speed monitoring equipment and sit out, recording the speeds of all vehicles and the details of those who are speeding. Some of the volunteers were the usual suspects, those who always turn out for their community, but there were enough new faces to remind me what a special village we lived in.

Through the efforts of our parish councils and elected representatives, and the support of those volunteers, Middle Barton was included in Oxfordshire County Council's pilot scheme to make all villages 20mph zones and, supported by data provided by Speedwatch volunteers, consultation for three possible traffic-calming buildouts has taken place. Objections to these measures seemed to come from older, well-off individuals who wanted to preserve the rural nature of the village. They certainly did not see themselves as part of the problem.

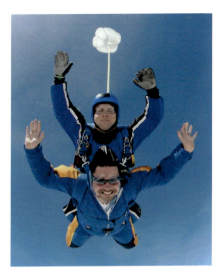

Taking to the skies for Ataxia UK, 2014

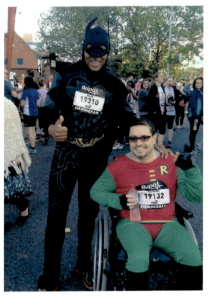

The Birmingham Half with Batman (Mark) 2014

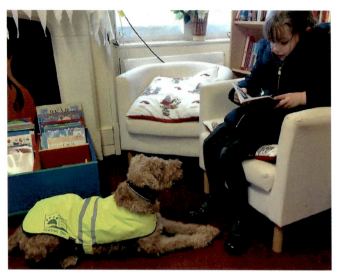

Tara the Reading Dog, 2017

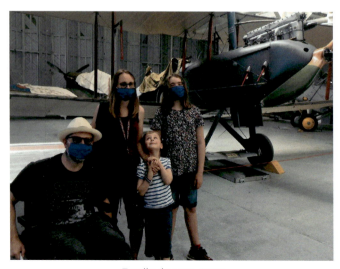

Family day out, 2020

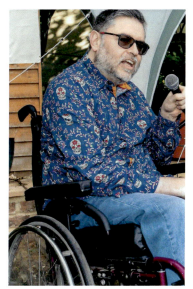

Letting loose, 2021

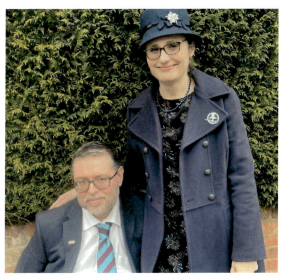

On the way to Windsor Castle, 2022

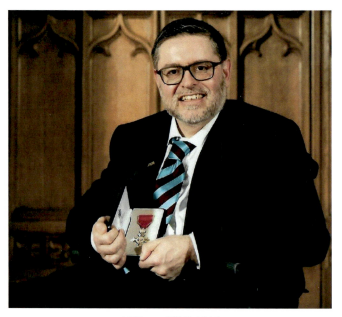

With my MBE, 2022

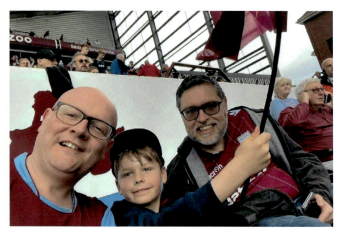

Billy's first Villa game (photo by Uncle Pat), May 2022

CONCLUSION: (JUST LIKE) STARTING OVER

Early retirement had suddenly given me the space and time I needed to pursue the things that were meaningful to me and not what our society promotes or rewards. I could develop the creativity that had always been with me: my love of representing people and storytelling. I started to realise that the meaning of life isn't about how much you earn, but about finding fulfilment and purpose.

I realised this is how I could become an Übermensch (superman) again. Not being bound by the moral rules (shame) and conventions of a capitalist society, following my own will to power (confidence), and overcoming myself to achieve excellence (meaning).

Volunteering enabled me to find, explore, and

develop my passions and understand a bit more about myself, and gave me a reason to fight. You can do what you love! How many jobs offer that? I have been volunteering now for as long as I worked, and have found it so much more fulfilling. I have been able to represent and support other people with ataxia, also encouraging them to become strong advocates and volunteers themselves. I have learned so much, made a valuable network of friends, and become part of another community. Each opportunity led me to others, and closer to finding meaning. Working with children emphasised the importance of good parenting. Primary schools are places for children to learn and grow, but the attitudes and behaviours they see at home will stay with them forever.

Working in my local community has been wonderful. There are many others who have literally driven those projects and put in hours of work alongside me. Good people who care about the place they live in. Getting to know them has been a privilege. There is real magic in coming together as a community to solve a problem. I think the unplanned, chaotic, imaginative, random nature of things that we do along the way are priceless.

Finding meaning has a price. Public services have been repeatedly slashed over the last 14 years of austerity; our National Health Service, police, education, local government, social care and criminal justice systems have been purposefully eroded to the point of collapse. All under the pretence of slashing welfare expenditure, upholding individual freedoms and promoting economic growth through free markets and trade. Charity and philanthropy do what they can to fill these gaps, and it feels really good to be partly responsible for a successful bus company, but communities doing everything themselves is not a viable long-term solution.

As much as helping other people is great, volunteering is a terrific form of self-care. The people I have met and the connections forged have made me feel better about myself than any difference I may have accomplished. Volunteering is like a garden. All you really need to volunteer is commitment and enthusiasm. It's best not to do it on your own. It is really hard work and making a success of it depends on how much effort you put in. It can quickly become unmanageable, lonely, and thankless. As with work, we need to keep moving as new networks and opportunities appear. Unlike work, it should always be on your own terms and fun.

Death once again loomed over my life. For me, it heightened the need to live in the present and the great importance in finding meaning in life. Then came the pandemic.

Part Five

Times Like These

The pandemic changed everything, especially intefering with my volunteering duties during lockdown. Ridiculous ups and downs occurred, but opportunities for community activism remained and my political awakening was starting.

LIVING IN A PANDEMIC: LOCKDOWN POLITICS

Do you recall your last normal day? On the 3rd of March 2020, I spent a day trapped in meetings in London where I retold a joke a bus colleague had made a day earlier. He'd reported a cough in one of our buses as 'Tucana virus'. Our first bus was a VW Tucana. I added flippantly that there was more chance of me being gunned down by a shark on a bicycle than dying from coronavirus. After that, the lockdowns started and my family and I rarely left our home. We did not leave our village for the next thirteen months.

I put the frightening speed that this situation overwhelmed the UK, and our lack of preparation, down to our misguided faith in, and the sluggish and inadequate response from, our government. Our government let us down because of how it chose to manage risk in combination with the entitlement, incompetence, and greed of its leadership. Populist neoliberal (Harvey, 2005) governments act on risk, towards protecting the wealth of a few, and seek to limit involvement of the state in everyday life because entrepreneurial initiative and private enterprise are seen as the keys to innovation and wealth creation. Such a weak response to a public health crisis, one that saw avoidable deaths (the Office for National Statistics report 170,000 excess deaths since the beginning of the 2020 lockdown) and wasted so much public money, is only to be expected from this kind of government. The pandemic held a blinding light to the weakened system we have. Austerity is a political choice; it opens the public health sector up to privatisation and ushers in the insurance model of social security (Clifford, 2020). The weak and the vulnerable are vilified and left to die alone. They are considered as noncontributors. Sadly, thanks to a right-wing media that promotes fear and division, this is on the watch of a government that people habitually vote for.

As neoliberal governments pursue a free market, involving ever more profit, they cut unprofitable but vital public services. The gap between the rich and the poor widens. In response to deep cuts that left our rural community without public transport, I helped set up and run a community transport service in 2016. Our volunteers and most of our passengers are mostly over 60. We support our local school and many groups. All of our volunteers are unpaid and are very proud of what we do. At the same time, we all resent that we have been left with no option but to take this action ourselves.

Today, the days of free university education that the baby boomers enjoyed are gone in England, Northern Ireland, and Wales. With more people than ever applying to university today, and racking up a lifetime of debt to do so, we should have the best politicians ever. Problem is, and this statement shouldn't surprise you if you've picked up this book, most senior politicians seem mediocre at best. They are what Italian economist Carlo M Cippola describes in his theory of 'stupid people' (Cippola, 2011). They are everywhere, in all walks of life, and their numbers and their sheer destructiveness is always underestimated. A stupid person is one who causes not only losses to themselves but also to other people. Equally dangerous are 'bandits.' Grifters and charlatans who, driven by self-interest, manage to achieve a benefit for themselves at the expense of everyone else. The current government seems to be full of stupid people and bandits, ready to manipulate people for their own gain.

The media plays a major role in stoking the fear and apprehension that enables this. For example, a report by the Migration Observatory in 2023 (The Migration Observatory, 2023) found that concerns amongst voters about immigration reached an all-time high of 48% in 2016. Politicians and the media resurrected this fear with 'small boats' at the end of 2023. Whistleblower Christopher Wylie, raised concerns that the EU referendum was won through fraud, accusing the campaigning organisation Vote Leave of improperly channelling money. Vote Leave was fined £61,000 after being found guilty of breaking electoral law during the Brexit campaign by the Electoral Commission (an independent body in the UK that regulates political financing). It's time to start asking why and challenge the actions of politicians. Grifters and charlatans in the government capitalised on this, as they would again during the pandemic. If I were to go into the government's abject failure in the UK's economy, transport, health and social care, environment, immigration, and public services, I'd need another book. These were some isolated examples to demonstrate the way people are manipulated, divided, and distracted by the government and the media. This must be understood in order to hold our government accountable for its actions.

Over the summer of 2021, I attended a public independent enquiry into the government's handling of the pandemic, chaired by a Queen's Counsel (an experienced senior barrister). Such an enquiry involved expert witnesses and politicians giving statements and being cross-examined under oath. Consequently, I know that the way this crisis has been handled by the government has been nothing short of deplorable. In my opinion, no direction or leadership was shown during the pandemic. Public money was wasted on defective PPE equipment, or siphoned through newly formed companies that won lucrative contracts through VIP lanes, with the consequence of letting Covid rip through our society. The outright profiteering of the private sector, especially utility companies, was yet to come...

That such an enquiry had to be put together by the public and wasn't attended by government ministers highlights our crisis of governance: its blatant lack of scrutiny and accountability. The sessions on the impacts of the government's handling of the pandemic on disabled people, who found that 'do not resuscitate' instructions had been placed on their notes, and frontline workers, who would be with people in their last moments when their families could not, were particularly harrowing.

From orbit to lockdown

My retirement from full-time work had already been a tremendous change. One which helped me to adapt to this one. When I retired in 2012 and left the busy lifestyle well behind me, I stopped wearing a watch. I was suddenly free to spend time on myself and my family. Although Helen teases sometimes that I am like an 'elderly shut-in', I did not find staying in a problem. I am fortunate to have a garden, yet finding the time to sit in the shade with a book is something I found harder to do over the last few summers before lockdown.

The first lockdown had a profound effect on my voluntary work. I had just been elected as co-chair of Ataxia UK. There was another candidate with ataxia who had a wealth of skills and experience that were quite different to mine. The best outcome for Ataxia UK would be if we worked together; I could work to my strengths and he to his. I also took inspiration from a friend who had championed the co-sharing of leadership roles.

Knowing that our business could absorb a lengthy suspension because of its low overheads, OurBus Bartons suspended services in March 2020. I had booked a daring wheelchair abseil from London's ArcelorMittal Orbit in July 2020. Much to Helen's relief, this didn't go ahead. Mine was a small event, but when you think of all the other events, large and small, that didn't go ahead that summer, it became a real problem for many charities. My co-chair at Ataxia UK and I had several meetings to figure out how to support our charity to adapt and survive.

Like many with ataxia, I did not receive a letter from the NHS confirming that I was a 'vulnerable person'. I think this was an oversight due to poor organisation and lack of planning, but it meant I already had to come out fighting. When supermarkets began to release delivery slots, a lot of disabled people who depend on deliveries were missed out. This happened to me, so to make sure I was included my brother, Ant, emailed Mike Coupe, CEO of Sainsbury's plc, with the email equivalent of 'Paddington's hard stare' and forwarded it to me so I could use it. I also filled in the government's list and soon received an email from Sainsbury's to say that my address had been passed to them by the government and matched up with their customer list. This meant that I would be able to book slots as a vulnerable customer. Shopping deliveries were limited: only available 72 hours in advance and you never knew if it would be cancelled or what was going to turn up in terms of substitutions of the items you actually ordered.

The issue of not being recognised as clinically extremely vulnerable (CEV) and included in the government's shielding scheme – which had prevented me from accessing home-shopping slots – returned with being overlooked for vaccination. Once again, I had to fight to correct it. After several requests to my GP, I was finally recognised as CEV and received my first vaccination as part of that group.

As the year dragged on, things got mentally hard for everyone. According to the Office for National Statistics (Office for National Statistics, 2020), the equivalent of 19 million adults in Great Britain reported high levels of anxiety during 2020. Refuge, the UK's largest domestic abuse charity, reported that in one week in 2020, the National Domestic Abuse helpline saw a 25% increase in calls and online requests for help (Refuge, 2020).

In a survey recently completed by Scope, 59% of disabled people reported feeling forgotten by the government and 41% expected their lives to get worse following the pandemic (Scope, 2020). This is disgraceful; we should be looking at ourselves and the way we live.

What should have been a relief and a glimmer of hope ... my first vaccination, just showed how shielding had affected my confidence. It was a cold day and I had to travel to a nearby town. As soon as we arrived, I started to feel anxious, being aware of the number of people. As soon as I transferred out of the car, my glasses steamed up. Unconfident of where I was and being unable to see, I let Helen push me to the entrance. The plan had been for me to do all this on my own as we had the kids in the car. But I didn't want to be left alone. As we entered the warm medical centre, my glasses steamed up again. A volunteer in a high-vis jacket with a clipboard stood above me and, highly unusually, spoke directly to me. I replied with a frightened whimper and, after that, Helen took charge. I was shocked that a confident person like me was reduced to this.

Masking up like the caped crusader

Negotiating this new world with a mask showed me how much I relied on smiling at people. It felt awkward not being able to do so. As most experts agree that between 70% and 93% of communication is non-verbal, that change must have been difficult for everyone. For me, I think smiling started as an unconscious way of warding off any 'unwanted helpers', but it is also a key signal to others when you catch that awkward glance and can return it with a big smile. I call it the 'everything's fine' smile; it can have a lovely mirror effect as people read my signal ('I'm one of you guys!') and smile back. Roald Dahl talks a lot about how his genuinely good characters smile with their eyes, such as the father in *Danny, the Champion of the World*. Whilst wearing a mask, I tried smiling with just my eyes – it didn't seem to have an effect. I also found that people avoided eye contact more than before. I suspect you need both your eyes and your mouth to smile!

I noted also that people had different views on wearing masks. Quite simply – if you can wear one, you should. If you don't, you are part of the problem. In my few trips out to local towns after the lockdowns, I estimated that about 60% of people wore masks in the street and about 90% in a shopping centre. I looked at anyone not wearing a mask and wondered why: did they have a hidden disability, were they facing anxiety, were they expressing their defiance or their God-given freedom of choice, did they leave theirs at home, were they carrying theirs in a pocket to put on when going into a shop? Probably a mixture of all these reasons. With the country neatly divided over every major issue, I wondered how many of those who decided they could not or would not wear a mask also voted to leave the EU. I admit I fell into a pattern of assuming they might be right-wing, flat-earthers, anti-vaxxers, conspiracy theorists, xenophobes, racists, and/or tabloid readers. I like to think I am a genuinely good person, with an open mind, and a supporter of a supportive society, so I resisted the urge to sigh, roll my eyes and shake my head. They may have seen the wheelchair, but did not know my reason for wearing a mask, as I didn't know theirs.

On my first trip out with my family, we went to Stratford. Feeling uncomfortable about being in a crowd, I was approached as usual by curious folks admiring my trike. But this time everyone said, 'Keep safe' as a farewell greeting. I'd never heard it said repeatedly by different people; the warmth, sense of shared hardship and genuine concern reminded me that other people are on my side. This helped me find the strength to put myself back out there over the coming months. So, thank you to you all.

Working from home

At the end of March 2020, I brought a professional membership on Zoom, the video chat platform. This meant events I hosted would not be limited to the forty minutes you're allowed on the free version. I opened a virtual pub, The Olde Sea Dogge (in honour of Tara), for my friends and I to catch up every Friday. A very touching moment was when a friend's wife came home from a nightshift at a supermarket. She popped in to say goodnight and was roundly applauded by everyone in the pub. As we acclimatised to this strange new version of a social life, our kids also adapted to learning and socialising on online platforms.

I tried online gaming. The only issue was that I often appeared in the midst of battle, and then while I was still looking around, somebody ran past and killed me. This dispiriting cycle continued for as long as I played! The auto-aim function didn't seem to work, stripping me of what little ability I had. I usually favoured a support role – a medic who followed the action, healing people. I tried meeting my brother online and chatted as we played *Battlefield 1*. Predictably our conversation was interrupted by sudden cries of 'Look out!', 'Ahh, I'm down!' or 'Go on without me!' Playing online is interesting and it's a really important social tool, yet it is the communal aspect of being part of a group that appeals to younger gamers. I'm just not convinced it's for me. My reactions aren't fast enough.

Online meetings were not the same as meeting face to face, but they made the world so much smaller and more accessible for me. Initially, I wanted to encourage my friends to meet up and to host my own meetings. I hadn't realised how meeting online would increase my sense of involvement and develop my own activism. I have attended so many online events here in the UK and globally. My new role as co-chair of Ataxia UK shifted seamlessly to online as, free from the need to travel, I found I had more opportunities to engage with staff.

Quickly adapting to the new virtual world, our brilliant staff team at Ataxia UK hosted online meetings for weekly discussions of TV shows, books and films, well-attended quizzes, branch meetings, yoga, pilates, mindfulness, and sessions with a speech therapist. With our last face-to-face conference in 2019, the team now organised successful online conferences. The InControl project saw the 'All About Ataxia' workshops increase to quarterly and be delivered online, attracting new volunteers. I was proud to see the last couple of workshops being run by these volunteers as they encouraged people to stand up for themselves and be assertive when dealing with others. A survey of our friends in 2022 evidenced that volunteering plays an important role in enhancing the wellbeing of the ataxia community. Volunteers engaging with Ataxia UK experienced increased wellbeing compared with those who did not volunteer.

During this early optimism and encouraged by the fundraising exploits of Captain Tom, I completed the 2.6 Challenge to fundraise at home – a nationwide event on the 26th of April 2020 that you could do anywhere. I completed 26 lengths of my garden path in 26 minutes. My path is only 8m long, however the gentle slope, the uneven paving slabs, the hard tyres of my wheelchair, and the time limit made it quite a challenge! I was also a guest on my first podcast, the subject of which was being a teenager with ataxia. Before we started, I introduced myself to the younger guests as 'the voice of experience' – Great Uncle Bulgaria if you will. As I said it, I remembered that young people don't necessarily know who Great Uncle Bulgaria is. I wondered if it would help if I explained his position in the Womble hierarchy but then quickly realised that would be pointless because they probably wouldn't know who the Wombles were! For those of us who do know ... 'Remember You're a Womble'!

A wise friend of mine said I would look back fondly on these days as an unexpected time to spend with our families. It reminded me of how John Lennon's 5-year break to be a stay-at-home dad marked the final stage in his journey of self-evolution. He had identified a cause he believed in and finally found the right people with which to share his happiness. It also reminded me of someone else I had been reading about. Christopher J. McCandless, who, at just 24, turned away from society and went to the Alaskan wilderness to look for the truth and answers within himself (Krakauer, 2011). He may have died a lonely death, but not before he realised that we alone are responsible for finding our own happiness and choosing who to share it with – as we know thanks to his journal. I agree with Chris. Happiness is not only to be found in the wealth and status of individualism, it is only real when shared. We all need to seek out the magic that can be found in working together as a community. I think volunteering can help you achieve this.

Black Lives Matter and Confirmation Bias

During that first UK lockdown, I could see how the lived experience of some disabled people was becoming the norm for others, and they didn't like it! To some, surviving on welfare benefits; rarely, if ever, going out; and going without was a totally unacceptable infringement of their human rights. The irony is that this is the fate to which our most vulnerable have been doomed for years.

My daughter's friends had a competition to see who could stay in bed and watch TV for the longest. Of course, that's just kids being kids, playing games as the norms of society fluctuated. But how easily the lived experience of some disabled people became a kids' game of endurance. For the first time in their lives, some of my non-disabled friends were facing real uncertainty with their finances and health. That made me realise how lucky I was that my position hadn't been shaken like others in my friendship group.

From the beginning of the pandemic, I could sense a fantastic opportunity emerging. I felt society had broken through many of the costly and archaic barriers to equality we had had to live with for years. I hoped that as people worked from home, they would be better able to understand themselves and provide the support that their children, elderly relatives, neighbours or friends really needed, and appreciate just how much damage we have done to our environment. This was a chance for humanity to come together, evolve, and revolutionise how we tackle global issues such as climate change, how we treat each other, and how to transform our toxic political system, media, and society.

When George Floyd was murdered by police in America, the public reaction highlighted the intersectionality between all oppressed groups. How discrimination is not a problem for one group, but a problem for all of us. Disabled people are not being murdered in the street, but hundreds have been murdered by the cruelty of the DWP. Bella chose to make a donation to Floyd's family, but the effects of his murder extended far into all our lives in 2020, especially into football. The games were still played. The grounds eerily empty. This summer was different in another way ... and no I didn't take to the streets to fight crime Batman-style. I'm still talking about football. Before each kick-off, the players of both teams would touch the ground with a knee, pause, and slowly rise to their feet in a gesture of solidarity with Black victims of racial inequality and police brutality around the world. This response to the Black Lives Matter protests was inspired by the much earlier protest of American football player Colin Kaepernick, who knelt during the American national anthem before a game in 2016 to protest against police brutality. This was almost four years before George Floyd was murdered by police and it ignited tensions around the world. Donald Trump and his Republican allies railed against this. At the end of that 2017 season, Kaepernick was released by his club and never played professionally again.

Aston Villa's Captain, Tyrone Mings, named alongside Greta Thunberg as one of Europe's young 'visionary leaders' in 2020 by *Forbes* magazine, led the campaign in the Premier League. It wisely kept away from the emotive national anthem. He was also part of a young England team that had qualified impressively for the European Championship. Also in that team was Marcus Rashford MBE who had repeatedly embarrassed the government by providing funds for them to tackle child poverty when it would not. Not only were they playing exciting football, this team were standing up for victims of discrimination on difficult ground. I strongly identified with them and wanted to show my support. To my horror, some supporters booed this gesture straight away. Sensing an opportunity to jump on the bandwagon, politicians on the right took the opportunity to pledge their support for the team, and also openly criticise 'taking the knee' as a political gesture that they felt had no part in the game. Some used a demonstrably false conspiracy theory to condemn Black Lives Matter as a shadowy, political moneymaking operation. This was institutional racism in action. In response, the players, the manager and ex-professionals had to explain that Black Lives Matter does not mean only that 'Black lives matter', it means 'all lives matter', but Black lives were especially endangered and needed everyone's support.

Taking a position on Black Lives Matter was pretty easy for me. I believe in equality of opportunity and an enabling supportive society founded on democratic principles. All lives matter, and in support of this we must recognise the cruelty that has been meted out specifically to Black people for centuries, ensure we reject racism in our lives and educate our children, friends and families by refusing to keep silent when we see it. Being 'woke' (alert to racial prejudice and discrimination) is just another way of saying you have empathy for others.

Racism is not the same as ableism – I think of them as close relatives. Our struggles are distinctly different too. A big difference between racism and ableism is slavery. The first slaves reached America in 1619. In Don Cornelius' Soul Train Nightclub in San Francisco in early 1974, comedian Richard Pryor told his audience a story about an everyday experience of racism, then he said, 'We've had 400 years of this shit.' The audience laughed. It was, and still is, part of their shared experience. The struggles of a person of colour has similarities with those borne by disabled people; we all know how it feels to be discriminated against.

Black Lives Matter challenged a lot of people. Both White supremacists and the kind of people who proudly say they don't see colour. Otto English (English, 2022) shows how much of the history we understand as being 'true' has been perverted to serve the needs of privileged, abled, White men. When these core beliefs are challenged, it creates cultural dissonance. Confirmation bias, the twisting of the facts (fake history), provides comfort and support and makes it go away. From one angle, this is how Twitter works. It is easy to stay in the echo chamber of our 'Following' tab and difficult to take a trip into the 'For You' tab, where Twitter's algorithm exposes us to some uncomfortable views that can trigger our own 'cultural dissonance.'

Confirmation bias explains how the government could produce a report (Commission on Race and Ethnic Disparities, 2021) into race inequality that suggested institutional racism is not really a problem, fuelling the clash between nationalism and Black Lives Matter that played out over the summer. Our elites did not want to be reminded that this country has a racism problem. In *Empireland: How Imperialism Has Shaped Modern Britain* (Sanghera, 2021), Sathnam Sanghera reminds us that while human behaviour and history is complex and nuanced, common behaviours persist. He explains that every nation believes it is exceptional and better than others, putting itself at the centre of the map. The British brand of exceptionalism is particularly strong because Britain has not been successfully invaded by a foreign army since 1688. We have never had to look carefully at ourselves after defeat, as most of our European neighbours have. After all, we were on the victorious side in both world wars, reinforcing the idea of the plucky British as stoic, proud survivors in the face of great hardship.

It isn't just racism this happens with. Facing down problems such as poverty, misogyny, homophobia, and ableism also creates dissonance. It explains the chronic under-reporting of the murder of Sabina Nessa, as the police were accused of not taking killings of women of colour seriously, or the government's pathetic promise to make the streets safer for women following the kidnapping and murder of Sarah Everard by a serving policeman that hadn't been vetted properly. Unsafe streets aren't murdering women, predatory men are. That is not something that much of the general public, the media, or politicians have empathy for or particularly want to address either. Institutional racism is just one of the structural issues currently underpinning our society.

What changed during the lockdowns?

Our home lives changed, still revolving around our brilliant kids: Billy (5) and Bella (10). Homeschooling was fun, although was at the limits of my knowledge trying to teach Key Stage 2 Maths. Helen is a maths teacher and was just about to start a new job. Fortunately, she was able to work from home for the first few months. We missed friends and family, but we had each other and had escaped Covid so far. Just before the lockdown began, we restored our garden trampoline, which our dog had mostly eaten, and our kids spent lots of time on that as the weather improved. They went out for bike rides most afternoons to keep active. I joined them sometimes. I had been inside a lot, so lost some of the activity I was doing. I increased the length of my workouts on the THERA-Trainer I had bought when I had retired to compensate. I took an instant and irrational dislike to Joe Wicks, the body coach who did PE classes on YouTube. Things were fairly quiet. The most danger I was in was when my wife used the dog clippers to cut my hair and hoovered me afterwards.

Soon, Helen had developed a real skill for cutting my hair. She gradually got faster and more confident. She even bought her own scissors, cape, and spray bottle. No more dog clippers for me! Shopping slots were always available, once on the list, and substitutions and shortages were minimal. I have not seen as many Villa matches on TV in my entire life as I did in that first lockdown year. The fact I watched them with my 6-year-old son was a bonus. You get used to the barrage of questions: can a goalkeeper be offside? Or what if the referee scores a goal? I took on homeschooling with him too. I enjoyed this unexpected time we spent together, counting with money and learning about Queen Victoria, whilst I became increasingly concerned that the Key Stage

2 Curriculum lacks balance and champions an unhealthy obsession with grammar over creativity.

Aware that Covid is airborne, OurBus Bartons bought a Steam generator that disinfected the air in the buses, so that we were able to restart a limited service in August 2020. We had to suspend it again at the start of 2021 for another 4 months. During this time, we helped individuals get to medical appointments, but I felt like we'd been abandoned. We introduced bookable and socially distanced seating, and made mask wearing compulsory. Then, in July 2021, all restrictions ended. I felt that throughout there had not been any trustworthy, coherent, or timely advice from the government; they were too busy partying.

Living through the pandemic majorly affected a lot of people. As lives changed forever, there was a lot of time to reflect. Spending so much time alone, people took the opportunity to reassess their lives, look at their regrets, and do something about them. The marriages of several friends fractured under this extra pressure. Better used to spending time together, our marriage held up. I identified a few building projects around our home and garden to get done when restrictions were lifted. Helen decided to become a rock star. She was playing an acoustic guitar and singing along most evenings. A school friend of hers became a professional songwriter and musician, and I think she always wondered what would have happened if she had taken this path too.

Maybe pebbles in the stream of life cannot change your destiny. I knew this was a pure expression of Helen's self, and wanted to do everything I could to support her. I bought her a Fender – signature Kurt Cobain Jaguar model. Actually my dream guitar. She already had an amp and cables. It snowballed from there! Pedals, microphones, speakers, and recording equipment. An important leap was to share her enthusiasm with other people. A friend and neighbour joined and started playing a bass guitar Helen retrieved from her parents' loft – later upgrading to a lovely instrument of her own. Bella joined as drummer and band artist, and The Jargonelles were formed.

Helen wrote her own songs – bleak and nihilist songs that would be at home in the '90s – and really enjoyed rehearsing and performing songs from her youth. The practices sounded like fun; I hear her laughing in such a natural way. Why didn't she find spending time with me that much fun? Of course, this wasn't about me, but about supporting Helen. Desperate not to be left out, I became the band's manager, although Helen dismissed most of my advice to play to the crowd and do sing-along songs they could dance to. I think Helen saw this as selling out! I'm so pleased that although it started as fun, Helen applied her drive to the band. She definitely 'bought a ticket!' The Jargonelles are very good and have played a few local gigs – the sky is the limit!

My idea of my self changed too. Still furious that Brexit had stripped me of my freedom of movement,

I applied to become an Irish citizen through my grandparents. It was a long-held plan. I had already gathered the necessary certificates to prove my grandparents were both born in Dublin and had married, and my father's documentation that proved he had married and had a son. With a year left on my British passport, I applied to be entered on the Irish Foreign Births Register in July 2020. It was announced soon after that the team that were processing these applications was being redeployed, and there was no estimate for when processing would continue. It only took two years.

AN MBE

While I was trying to make sense of pandemic lockdown politics, I was contacted in late November 2020 to ask if I would accept an MBE in the coming New Year's Honours list. It was two years after I had initiated the nomination, so I was surprised and delighted. I accepted straight away. When letting my family know and the people who had supported my nomination, they were sworn to secrecy until the lists were published. Of course, I used that time to completely overthink it. For the next few weeks, as I awaited the official announcement, I could feel my own mortality breathing down my neck. When you are constantly pushed to the edge of society, you question your own achievements.

I was reading *A Promised Land* by Barack Obama (Obama, 2020) at the time and could understand the unwelcome pressure he felt to be an inspiration as the first Black president of the US. Being the first person with Friedreich's ataxia to be awarded such an honour was great, but I didn't want to be an 'inspiration' either. It is a lazy trope that is often used to put pressure on other disabled people whose impairments make it difficult or impossible to interact with the world as it is: 'He can do it, why can't you?' I have not overcome my disability; as earlier chapters of this book have shown, I have adapted to my impairment and performed consistently at a high level for more than twenty years. I have struggled through a decade in the 'normal' world and managed to survive: I bought a ticket and have been lucky enough to overcome *some* of the barriers that society places against people with disabilities. Now, like Obama, I felt the need to work to dismantle those same barriers for other disabled people. I wanted my story to be a boost to others who have to put in extra work and effort to achieve their goals. I will only tolerate being called an inspiration by people with the same condition as me. Even within my condition, progression can make that comparison unfair.

What Obama did to change the discriminatory structure was to promote people from backgrounds like his. In his first term as president, Obama nominated Sonia Sotomayor as a Supreme Court Justice – only the third woman, the first woman of colour, the first Hispanic, and the first Latina to serve the Supreme Court. For Obama, she is someone with 'intelligence, grit and adaptability' who has had to work harder to succeed due to her ethnic background. His endorsement struck a chord with me. I could not promote or employ disabled people myself, but I could help educate and encourage them to seek out new skills and opportunities. Especially through the InControl project with Ataxia UK, in which we were encouraging volunteers with ataxia to develop their skills to help run Ataxia UK.

As 2020 finally drew to a close, like many others, I didn't know what to expect from the future as the big news – at least for me – was announced. I'd agreed to have my contact details shared with the media. I didn't think anyone would notice. I was pleasantly surprised when word spread. New Year's Day 2021 was like a birthday. My phone did not stop ringing; friends and colleagues who I hadn't spoken with in years reached out to give their congratulations, as well as deliveries of cards, letters, and bottles of champagne. I was touched that one of my friends had spotted my name in *The London Gazette* and called to congratulate me.

My citation in *The London Gazette* read: 'Co-Chair of Ataxia UK For services to People with Disabilities and to the community in Middle Barton, Oxfordshire.' This sentence represents more than 20 years of my life: home study, university, my career, my association with Ataxia UK, my wider voluntary work, and how they all came together to benefit other people. I had made it very clear throughout my application that I did not want to get caught up in the 'triumphing over adversity' narrative again.

An MBE is an order of knighthood, as it is not one of the top two of five – I'm not Sir Richard (yet!). Awarded by the monarch or a member of the royal family, the medal itself is usually presented within a few months at Buckingham Palace or Windsor Castle. I hoped mine would be presented by Prince William so that we could talk about our beloved Aston Villa! As a Member of the Order of the British Empire, I am entitled to wear the medal, use the letters 'MBE' after my name, book a chapel at St Paul's Cathedral for the weddings of my children and their children, and commission my own coat of arms. I see it as a recognition of my work. It is a point of entry into the establishment also. I soon found that people behaved differently with me. People don't interrupt me in online meetings anymore! My first official act was to write to the DWP to insist that when they contact me in future, it was to be with my full title. I knew they wouldn't, but it felt good. These were little things for me; not the real prize, which is in the good I can do going forwards.

I do not feel humbled, I feel honoured. And, as always, our kids can be relied on to keep me grounded. Billy explained helpfully that 'Mr Bean got a medal from the Queen for rescuing her dog.' Bella added that it was: 'Quite good.' In the long run, it took an incredible amount of hard work, sacrifice, perseverance, a little luck, and lots of support to get there. It is an achievement in which I acknowledge all of my friends, family, and colleagues. I am so grateful to them all. But it is my wife to whom I owe the most. This award must have been a bittersweet reminder of all the unconditional support she had given and the sacrifices she had made for me over the years. She raised me up. It wouldn't have happened without her. Thankfully, she knows it is her achievement just as much as mine. In an interview on Radio Oxford, trying to explain exactly when things changed for me, I said: 'It was when I met my current wife' instead of 'It was when I met my future wife.' Making it sound as if I planned to have other wives! As well as putting up with my terrible neediness, she has been part of everything good that has happened to me since we met.

Even though I had initiated the process, it was by no means a foregone conclusion. I found out quite a bit of investigation had taken place. Those who had nominated me were interviewed at length and sworn to secrecy. Like every occasion during lockdown, it was odd not being able to celebrate properly with friends and family. A few months later, the royal warrant arrived sealed in a tube – one of the last to have been signed by Prince Phillip and the Queen together. I love its archaic wording: 'By the grace of God, Her Majesty the Queen bestows this Honour on our trusty and well beloved Richard Christopher Brown Esquire.' As the investiture ceremonies had stopped for the pandemic, my fears of a sudden death resurfaced. I hoped I would live to have my day at the palace.

Too real for TV

I decided the best way to make the most of my new profile and change how the world sees disabled people was to be through the media of television. The *Ranganation* is a BBC2 current affairs comedy show with a panel of members of the public (and Romesh Ranganathan's mum) discussing the events of the last week with Romesh, celebrity guests, and a live audience. The show was being made via Zoom. As self-appointed 'King of Zoom', I applied to be on the panel. I wondered if my MBE might pique their interest. It did and an audition via Zoom was arranged that week.

The application I had to complete first asked about my burning passion, most embarrassing moment, and pet hate. Wide-open jumping-off points to show my personality. I talked about my passion for volunteering, but was careful to acknowledge the excellent support that has always made the difference. Keen to avoid the 'inspirational disabled person' trope, I hope I came across as a unique, modest, and interesting person. I confessed that my most embarrassing moment was taking a briefcase to school when I was 12. This was in the late-'80s, when having the right sports holdall to carry your books was quite a thing. I understood briefcases to be a symbol of organisation and professionalism. Wanting badly to convey both, and perhaps wanting to be like my public school cousins, I decided to buy one from Argos and take it to school. Big mistake. Being different when you're a teenager is good, but this was too much. It was 20 years before 'briefcase wanker' was made famous by *The Inbetweeners*, so I was ahead of my time! I should get my legal team to check if I am owed any royalties.

When it came up in the audition, I was ready. I explained how I'd recently asked my old school friends on Facebook if they remembered my briefcase, secretly hoping that I'd imagined it or maybe they had all forgotten. No chance. They all remembered. It got a laugh from the researcher and I was pleased that I had shown that I could take being laughed at and how I had turned an awkward teenage episode into an amusing anecdote about memory. I knew I had to be very careful with my pet hates. I know that outsider viewpoints aren't popular and I should definitely avoid getting on my soapbox and talking about access, ableism, or poverty. I had attempted to dismiss the question on my application by explaining being angry is pointless and something I try not to do. In the audition, the interviewer sensed I was holding back, 'But there must be something that makes you angry?' Under pressure to show some passion, I replied that social injustice makes me extremely angry. Then the floodgates opened! I spoke out about austerity, Brexit, Trump, and Covid. I think I mentioned social justice five or six times. I even mentioned disability and how the very common level of ignorance held by most people makes me despair.

I was concerned that my outburst had made me

look preachy and woke, but then they were looking for passion. I knew the key here was to keep things light, quirky, and funny. Maybe I should have just asked why the shower suddenly goes from very hot to very cold or why people in TV commercials behave unrealistically. Questions the Curious Orange from TMWRNJ might ask. We went on to talk about lockdown life, homeschooling, and Zoom meetings – all things I had crafted into anecdotes and touched on as humorous observations in my blog. I thought I'd turned it round at this point and the audition went well overall. I was surprised and a little disappointed not to be called back later that week. But as Colin Kaepernick says in the excellent *Colin in Black and White* (TV mini series, 2021): 'Rejection is not failure, it's a calibrator. It can help you learn who you are and what you want.'

Life carried on. When I caught an episode from the new series of *The Ranganation* a few months later, I noticed they had kept many of the same contributors as before: Glam Gran, Dogfather, Wheeler Dealer, Lord Dave, Oxbridge, and Romesh's mum. I realised that if the producers felt that they were close to a winning formula, it was one-in, one-out, there was serious competition for places. *The Ranganation* discussed a recent poll on Twitter which had asked people to choose who would be the best prime minister between Boris Johnson and Sir Keir Starmer. I would have gone in hard. Firstly, Boris Johnson was already prime minister, so we were being asked the wrong question. The question should have been: 'Do you think Boris Johnson is doing a good job as prime minister? Secondly, both have proved unfit for their jobs. As prime minister, Johnson's main jobs were to avoid deaths and act with integrity, diplomacy, and grace. Starmer's job was to form a credible opposition. Both have failed – Johnson catastrophically so. I don't think this observation would have gone down well on what is a light-hearted, current affairs show. The discussion soon turned to which of the two to go for a drink or on holiday with and touched on Johnson's (carefully manufactured) loveable, bumbling nature. This rambling conversation continued for almost nine minutes.

Following this, a new panellist was unveiled: a circus-trained acrobat. Undoubtedly highly skilled and with lots of funny stories, her selection made it clear to me that my activism wouldn't have fitted in. Romesh engages with the banter and then delivers a witty conclusion. It's his show; he is the smartest, funniest one – the king of the discussion. He ended this one with the observation: 'Neither are particularly inspiring; both look like they would have been kicked out of the apprentice by week three.' Not the scorching outspokenness I was hoping for from a fellow admirer of the great comedian Richard Pryor. Perhaps that was as far as Romesh and the writers on the show felt they could go on BBC2. I decided that I would be better at writing for TV rather than being on it! Something had awakened in me.

The Spencer Steadman Trust

My skills and experience proved useful again as I helped set up an educational trust in my cousin's memory. From agreeing on what the charity would do, to signing documents, and coordinating gala events, everything was done online. Apart from Kate, Spencer's wonderful sister, I didn't know the other seven trustees. As we began work in early 2020, the pandemic began to bite, but we carried on meeting up amidst hectic work or family lives – some calling in from around the world. I felt like a bit of an outsider at first. The others knew Spencer from public school and were definitely people I would never have met or worked with. They were all incredibly kind and loyal to Spencer's memory. We agreed to set up a trust in his name to support children from disadvantaged backgrounds to enjoy the opportunities that Spencer had. This turned out to be quite a challenging task during a pandemic. Eighteen months and many more meetings later, we had registered The Spencer Steadman Trust as a charity, opened a bank account, and identified several worthy projects to work with.

In 2021, the trustees met up in Regent's Park for the second anniversary of Spencer's death. Although I had seen many of them at the funeral, I was so happy to finally meet my new friends properly. We launched the charity at a gala dinner and auction at the English Speaking Union in Mayfair. Spurred on by this success, we held events at the House of Commons and at the House of Lords the following years. It was a pleasure to meet our first bursary students there – to hear about their difficult backgrounds and how the trust had helped them. Thanks to the generosity and commitment of Spencer's family and friends who attended, provided auction items, and made bids and donations, the trust has allocated almost a quarter of a million pounds to support students from lower socio-economic backgrounds. It also showed me that great meaning could still be found in online voluntary work.

One for all and all for one: Our community pub

During the lockdowns in the UK, it was still possible to coordinate some meaningful community action. Surprised to learn that the most recent tenants had left our village pub at the beginning of July 2021, and sure that there was plenty of interest within the community to intervene, I hosted a public meeting via Zoom to discuss the possibility of transforming The Fox Inn into a community pub. It had been a very difficult time for pubs. According to Campaign for Real Ale (CAMRA), 18 pubs close every day, but there are now 120 community-owned pubs with more on the way. Because they are owned by the community and their use of volunteers, they are exceptionally resilient and continue to have a 99% success rate. There are grants and plenty of advice available.

An MBE

The Fox Inn at Westcote Barton was an important part of our village, having been a busy pub for hundreds of years. It has been languishing in private ownership since 2000, bled dry for profit and burdened with debt. There had been a high turnover of tenants and the pub had often been closed for significant periods in the ten years I had lived in the village. A multinational hospitality company, Stonegate Group, registered in the Cayman Islands, absorbed the previous owner, Enterprise Inns, in 2020. The business model of tying tenants to a single supplier drains as much as 97% of turnover of a thriving pub. This had not worked well for our village pubs in the past.

Whilst we were fortunate to have other resources within our community, The Fox Inn was worth saving. It had furthered the social wellbeing and social interests of the community. It had been used for community events and meetings, as a venue for live music and for drinking and dining, and provided employment opportunities for people locally. It was popular with all sectors of the community, especially families at weekends. At lunchtimes, it attracted custom from local businesses, including Alpine F1 (formerly Renault F1) based nearby. Recent tenants sought to use locally sourced products for their menu, giving a much-needed boost to local markets.

Our first meeting agreed to move ahead and register The Fox as an 'Asset of Community Value' (ACV) with West Oxfordshire District Council. This sent a clear message to the owners and potential tenants that this community wanted to see a successful and well-run village pub and that the community's future support was conditional upon this. If it were to be put up for sale in the future, the community would have six months to put in a bid to purchase it. An ACV would also offer additional protection in planning terms should The Fox be the subject of a 'change of use' application by the owner.

Over the next couple of weeks, I went online and collected a considerable amount of testimony from villagers. I was reminded that in 2012, The Fox was awarded CAMRA's Oxfordshire 'Pub of the Year.' I found that 154 locals had signed an online petition asking the owners (Enterprise Inns) to keep the then current tenants in The Fox, as they were fulfilling its potential as a real asset to the community. Many also left heartfelt comments in support. 'Protect Our Fox' was formed on the 4th of August 2021, with me as chair and Helen as secretary, to apply for ACV status. The necessary signatures of 27 local residents were collected one by one over a weekend and, along with relevant information from the Land Registry, we sent it all off. Our application went to the Legal Team at West Oxfordshire District Council. As they are terribly understaffed, progress was painfully slow.

With the ACV in place, the new tenants were busy turning The Fox's fortunes around at the start of 2023. We were hopeful that Stonegate would finally invest the time, effort, and money needed to bring The Fox Inn up to a high standard. That June, amidst spiralling corporate debt, they informed those tenants of their intention to sell. Another example of the failure of the private sector. Our committee had just six months to set up a company, recruit a celebrity, commission surveys, hold events, manage publicity and crowdfund the money we needed to 'Save Our Fox.'

Our Bus Family CIC

Not everything turned out the way I hoped. In 2018, I set up Our Bus Family CIC (Community Interest Company) – a not-for-profit body aiming to support other communities in Oxfordshire and the UK, who, facing cuts to public transport, wanted to establish their own community transport operations using the OurBus Family umbrella. I hoped that this would remove a lot of the red tape that my colleagues and I had to negotiate to start our own bus company. OurBus Family would offer a ready-made corporate structure, policies, publicity, logos, and our experience, expertise, support and contacts. The idea was to support other communities by helping them apply for or raise their own start-up capital.

I met with several interested communities who had lost their bus services and spoke at a meeting of Oxfordshire Parish Transport Representatives at County Hall in Oxford. However, it soon became clear that we had underestimated other communities' desire to develop their own bus companies; they wanted us to set up and run one for them. Our ethos is volunteer-led and provides a light touch, but this did not seem to appeal to other communities, who would need to put in the extra work themselves. Another problem was that with no capital of our own to lend or give, we had nothing to offer beyond the prospect of hard work.

Despite being a CIC and repeatedly reporting as being dormant, HMRC chased us for paper tax returns every year. After four years of admin charges and a fine for a late return, my fellow directors and I finally dissolved the company at the end of 2021. We were charged an administration fee for that too! Just eighteen months later, OurBus Bartons would, once again, lead the way for other communities with its new electric buses.

For love: My investiture

Just over a year after the formal announcement of my MBE, restrictions had begun to ease and I received a letter summoning me to Windsor Castle. Because of the pandemic, recipients were only allowed one guest and there would be no refreshments available. I didn't mind, and was just relieved to be going at last. I did ask if I could bring a second guest to help me over the difficult terrain. The Investitures Office politely declined, explaining that they would make sure I was able to park at the castle itself and have a member of staff ready to help me.

An MBE

Before attending, I was frequently asked who would be performing the ceremony. St James's Palace can't say in advance so it is a complete surprise on the day. I wore a claret and blue striped tie in case it was Prince William, also an Aston Villa fan. I even wondered if it might be HM The Queen, as it was her Platinum Jubilee. The dress code seemed straightforward enough: a lounge suit or morning suit (no top hat though!) for men, and a dress and jacket for ladies. However, it was 'preferable' for ladies to wear a hat – I had read somewhere that the Queen prefers ladies to wear hats. Now, Helen doesn't like being told what to do, so I was a little concerned. I needn't have been. She looked absolutely fantastic in her cloche hat and navy-blue outfit, carefully chosen to match my suit. As a nice touch, she wore the necklace her granny had worn when she met the Queen in the '80s. She also wore a *Hunger Games* brooch as a symbol of defiance!

Security at Windsor Castle was tremendously tight. Armed police officers checked our invitations and IDs, while others checked under the car. While we sat waiting, Helen accidently pressed the horn. In that anxious moment, my first thought was that we were going to die in a hail of bullets. My second thought was that our car horn is so pathetic that we were more in danger of being laughed at. We were directed to a courtyard to park. The afternoon sky had darkened, promising rain. One of the many smartly dressed paiges showed us inside and accompanied us in a lift. I have never been congratulated and called 'Sir' so many times in one day! We were given programmes and a metal loop was attached to my lapel. We waited in the Queen's drawing room with about 20 other guests, paintings by Holbein, Van Dyck, and Rubens lining the walls.

It was going to be Princess Anne! A large video screen showed a previous investiture conducted by the princess. Recipients and guests were briefed on what to do. There were only 58 recipients that day, half the usual number. We were organised into a queue and shuffled down to a room adjoining the grand reception room, where the investitures were taking place. We could hear the army's string orchestra playing a mixture of classical and classic rock music. I watched the proceedings with interest, my anxiety increasing when I saw that every recipient spent a couple of minutes chatting with her. *What on earth have I got to say to her*? I thought. It was times like these that you had to try: 'You gotta buy a ticket.'

When it was my turn, I removed my face mask. Helen and I were separated. I waited at the edge of the brightest and most richly decorated room I have ever seen and saw Princess Anne chatting with the person who, just a moment ago, was waiting in the queue in front of me. I swelled with pride as the Lord Chamberlain read out my citation, 'Mr Richard Christopher Brown Esquire MBE, for services to Disabled People and the Community of Middle Barton in Oxfordshire.' The paige pushed me in my chair towards The Princess Royal and stepped back. I bowed my head. As Princess Anne attached the medal to the hook on my lapel, I thanked her and explained that I'd met her as a volunteer when she had opened the Soldiers of Oxfordshire Museum in Woodstock in 2014. She smiled and said, 'Such a lovely place. I keep meaning to go back, but never have time.' I was pleased we had established our conversation on Oxfordshire. She skilfully asked, 'Is Middle Barton very close to Woodstock?' I was impressed. Instead of glibly asking me, 'What do you do?', she had been well briefed and knew exactly why I was there and what I'd done. I was relieved to know that I was in the hands of a very experienced conversationalist. Anyone who has watched *The Crown*, a TV series based on the royal family, won't be surprised about this.

We continued to talk about my voluntary work. It was obvious that The Princess Royal had been briefed about OurBus Bartons. She said it was a wonderful service, but joked 'The wheels can fall off if you don't have the right volunteers.' I smiled and replied, 'We're unique and we do it for love, but there just aren't enough of us, are there, Ma'am?' She nodded and smiled knowingly. Our conversation moved to my work with Ataxia UK. 'Ataxia is such a difficult diagnosis; was Ataxia UK there for you at that time?' she asked. Once again, I was impressed that she already knew about my work with Ataxia UK. I explained that they were there for me when I was ready for them, and I was very grateful. I explained that I had made it my mission to be there for others going through their diagnosis. When she thanked me for all my work, it felt genuine.

That was it, I'd done it! The paige reappeared behind me, I bowed my head again and was returned to Helen who said it looked like I had to be dragged away! The string orchestra started playing the twirling melody of 'Clocks' by Coldplay. I gave the orchestra a big grin as I went past. In the next room, the medal was put in a box and handed back to me. Then, as cameras aren't allowed anywhere in state buildings, we had some professional pictures taken. We had a quick look at some of the collections of arms and armour and were shown outside to take a few selfies. It had rained softly while we were inside. It was such a slick operation; from start to finish we were only there for just over two hours.

It was an unusual, but very special day. I felt terrifically proud and was so glad that Helen was there to share it with me. As we left for our dinner reservations at Heston Blumethal's restaurant, we drove past Saint George's Chapel and I remembered my first visit to Windsor Castle as a child with Auntie Angela. I never imagined that this place would become part of my story one day.

THE PANDEMIC IS NOT OVER

I do not consider the Covid pandemic to be over. We've just entered a new stage, that's all. Although restrictions were lifted in April 2021 and my last lockdown post was in May 2021, I kept shielding until I had my second vaccination, by which time I had been shielding for thirteen months.

A huge proportion of the UK's Covid deaths are amongst disabled people. Through its disastrous mismanagement of the pandemic, this government has abandoned disabled people and their families, leaving them to experience hardship across all areas of life: increasing mental distress, social isolation and loneliness, food poverty, financial difficulties, workplace discrimination, problems accessing healthcare, and unequal access to medicine, vaccines, and social care.

In January 2022, I tweeted about my teacher wife

having to provide her own air filtration equipment for her classroom. The post caught on and received 5,000 likes, 1,390 retweets and 243k views. Once again, I made it sound like I had multiple wives.

Business as usual?

After months of being afraid and excluded, restrictions were lifted and lockdowns were forgotten. Disabled people had barely been mentioned in communications from the government during the UK's lockdowns and the spread of pavement cafes meant that city centres became no-go areas for disabled people. How did they expect us to navigate around these obstacles? As soon as office work became an inconvenience for ableds, a solution was quickly found. Working from home, which was beneficial to everyone, came under pressure from billionaire property owners and others with an interest in screwing commuters for profit. The decision to return to work was meekly backed by the government. As people were forced to return to the workplace, the dangerous gaps in accessing care at home exposed in 2016, and were not fixed then, were appearing once more.

I stepped down as co-chair of Ataxia UK in October 2021, after serving the maximum eight years as a trustee. My schedule felt empty. Despite being fully vaccinated, the complete lack of mitigations in schools made it impossible for me to return with any confidence as a voluntary reader. My son's interest in football, Aston Villa's eventual return to the Premiership in 2019, and the promise of an exciting future for the club convinced me that it was time to bestow the great honour of supporting Aston Villa upon him. My brother and I took him to his first game at Villa Park in May 2022. He was unusually quiet. I had expected to be subjected to a constant barrage of questions – I think he was overwhelmed by all the noise and excitement and slept in the car for most of the way back. For better or worse, Aston Villa have chosen him now. There might be dark and frustrating times ahead, but perhaps some trophies and a strong sense of identity and belonging will help him in life as they've helped me.

Trying to get back out there, we went to see Pearl Jam at Hyde Park Calling in July 2022. I looked around sadly at the mostly empty disabled area during the anthem 'Alive', remembering the strength that audiences had joined in in previous years, and thought, *But we aren't still alive, are we*? A slight amendment here: we were on ground level and Helen tells me there was a tier of wheelchair users behind us.

Another sign that our lives were opening up again was that my Irish citizenship was finally approved in November 2022. I had applied through my father's mother, Frances. Her maiden name was Walsh. I noticed my entry on the Irish Foreign Births Register was signed by an 'N. Walsh', a distant relative perhaps? I was a dual-national at last. Although it is only a piece of paper, I felt different. I had got my EU rights back, I was suddenly an interested observer of the unfolding nightmare, with the option to escape the UK if needed. I applied for my Irish passport immediately and it arrived a month later.

The biggest crossover in my volunteering experience was with the National Lottery. In 2019, they funded the InControl project, enabling Ataxia UK to connect with our community and recruit many volunteers through the lockdowns. It was so successful, there are plans to expand the brand to provide more information to enable people to take control of their lives. Ataxia UK recently received funds to continue the program and develop new strands around useful 'life hacks' and mental health.

In September 2021, I submitted an outline proposal to the National Lottery for £185,000 to purchase our first electric bus. The National Lottery liked it and we launched our 'Going Green' campaign at our local primary school the following February. The younger pupils had prepared some brilliant artwork and the older pupils spoke eloquently about the importance of protecting our environment to our assembled friends. We used this momentum to work up our stage two proposal, casting ourselves very much as outliers once again – that we were still the only voluntary operation of its kind in Oxfordshire and would be the first to go electric.

Our stage two proposal developed the complex practical elements of the project that I just hadn't considered. How would charging work? Where would we get the buses serviced? To answer these questions to the satisfaction of the National Lottery, we had to secure the land for, and build, our first depot. Helen's mum, Sue, helped us draw up a legal agreement to lease an area of land from the generous local farmer who had always allowed us to park our vehicles on his land. Luckily, our current garage was already servicing similar vehicles. As we gathered quotes, it became clear that we could purchase two electric, accessible buses from China for the price of one from Britain. Dependent on deliveries from the EU, British suppliers could not guarantee a price nor the amount of time needed for delivery. Remembering the passion that the children from our village school had shown for the environment, and how thousands of similar vehicles are being used by Amazon and DPD, we took the Chinese option and reworked our bid to make our operation fully electric. Once again, Martin, along with the rest of the team, put in a lot of work to secure the electric infrastructure we needed and was heavily involved throughout the manufacture of the buses, making sure that they were right for us. Similar to when we started, there were no figures available; we just had to make the best guesses we could with the knowledge we had. After a year of careful information gathering, the National Lottery accepted our bid and are very excited about playing a role in our amazing story. The pupils of our village school named the buses 'Basil Bus' and 'Lightning' and we are expecting to take delivery of them by mid 2024.

In November 2023, OurBus Bartons was a Bronze Award Winner in The Bus and Community Category of The 2023 UK Bus Awards. I spoke to them over the previous summer and gave them lots of information about our pioneering bus company, but they explained that their focus was on the national industry and the big players, so perhaps we should look at something better suited to the size and background of our operation. I was surprised when they called the bus hotline six months later to tell us that the awards ceremony had just taken place and that we had won an award. The other winners in our category were Stagecoach and Arriva – the former couldn't make a service through our village work in 2016. We had shown everyone that we, the community, could. It was a vindication of our efforts and a lovely Christmas present for all of our volunteers who had worked so hard.

CONCLUSION: TIMES LIKE THESE

The pandemic changed everything. The first year was intense. It exposed the widespread corruption, incompetence, and lack of ethics of our government. Whilst I experienced great fear and uncertainty as I struggled to fit myself into the newly created role of 'clinically extremely vulnerable', these times also provided unexpected benefits. I enjoyed homeschooling my 6-year-old son, and the virtual meetings and virtual socialising were great as they came without the hours of travelling and without the visual stigma of being a wheelchair user. I rekindled my love of film, music, and books. I found great comfort in listening to the Adam Buxton podcast, his rambling chats with celebrities and virtual hug at the end of each episode really helped me get through, as did my new friendship with Georg, an exceptional person and fellow ataxian.

Although I had to stop some of my voluntary work, I was still able to find meaning and make a difference. I became much more involved with Ataxia UK, helped get the Spencer Steadman Trust up and running, and worked with my community to protect our village pub. Receiving my MBE was an honour; it gave me some of my confidence back and a strong desire to use it to help others. OurBus Bartons had adapted and survived and returned to a full timetable in January 2022.

We all changed. Seeing such political dysfunction awoke a new sense of awareness within me. I had hoped that just surviving these times would make us realise how damaging our lives were for the planet. The global shutdown that emptied our roads and skies only saw CO_2 levels drop to 2006 levels. Our politicians and industries need to do much more. Hopes of a general empathy for others facing discrimination appeared with the Black Lives Matter movement but were quickly stamped out.

Since restrictions have been lifted, the government has just stubbornly doubled down on its irresponsible approach, sending children and teachers into schools that are unsafe, ending the vaccination programme and continuing to dismantle the NHS and other public services. There seems to be an obsession with denial, as people try to return to normal. Covid is not over. The pandemic is still ongoing and is a mass-disablement event; people with long Covid are being forced to reassess their

Conclusion: Times Like These

place in a woefully inadequate ableist, capitalist society.

The government has used Brexit and the pandemic to further increase the gap between rich and poor. Our essential workers are simply not valued by this government. They are woefully underpaid, unequipped, on zero-hour contracts or are saddled with debt. Many are now on strike for better pay and conditions.

As the first victims of austerity and the UK's 'hostile environment', disabled people have been warning this was coming for years. The government champions privilege whilst continuing to erode our civil rights. Much of the UK media has fed upon sensationalism and created panic and division, while enabling corruption to go unchallenged. But worse, we are starting to see narratives about disabled people being a financial drain on society. This government and the mainstream media have completely failed.

In June 2022, a public enquiry was set up to examine the UK's response to and impact of the pandemic, especially disparities within the seven protected groups under the Equalities Act (2010). We would finally know why 6 in 10 (59.5%) of all deaths involving COVID-19 for the period to July 2020 (27,534 of 46,314 deaths) were amongst disabled people (Office for National Statistics, 2020). Under the Inquiries Act (2005), the enquiry can compel the production of documents and call witnesses to give evidence on oath. This seemed to cause quite a panic amongst politicians unused to accepting accountability, as meeting notes, work diaries and mobile phone records were requested. Ongoing at the time of writing, the enquiry has already shown that the severity of the pandemic was greatly increased by the incompetence of the politicians leading the UK's response.

Feeling close to death is not unusual for disabled people. We have found ourselves in an increasingly hostile environment since 2010. Huge swathes of our media have normalised the hatred and suspicion of disabled people, and other minorities, for years. Many were also concerned that a post-Covid world would see disabled people as burdens once again. Austerity has given me an enemy to fight against and disabled people are my people to fight for.

Surrounded by death, I glimpsed hope. In the next part, I consider hope, take an overdue look at myself, suggest how we can change the world around us, and how we can live with our impairments.

Part Six

Gimme Some Truth

As restrictions were eased, I began to realise that it wasn't just traditionally marginalised groups like mine that were in trouble now, but pretty much everyone. My understanding of disability reached a good level. I became painfully aware that as oppressed people our rights had been seriously eroded by the government since 2010 and trampled on during the pandemic. I had always understood the importance of representation form my time as a student, but now I found I had a lot of opinions and a cause to fight.

BECOMING AN ACTIVIST

It started with a blog. I was offered the opportunity to submit a regular blog by Ataxia UK. I was convinced that between updating some pieces I had already written, and taking inspiration from my recently increased use of Twitter (now known as X), I would have no problem writing a modest target of 1,500 words a month. Blog posts don't need to be larger than that (they do for Google algorithms unfortunately). It meant I could keep writing regularly. After thinking about it, as a long-standing trustee of Ataxia UK, I wanted my views to be independent from those of the charity, so I decided to put them online.

I started 'World According to Me' at the end of 2018. On it, I write about my personal experience of life with ataxia and these posts are sometimes shared by the charity. I also go a bit deeper and write about wider social issues from my unique perspective as a disabled person. There is something in all of us that is curious and covetous. I have always wanted to show others how clever I was and how refined my tastes were. That may have been a misjudgement on my part! In the mid-'90s, I had a website that carefully listed my hobbies and interests. Let's face it, pages took so long to load back then, a list without pictures was ideal. With the important addition of sharing my experiences with the wider disability community, my blog serves that purpose today. There are perhaps more photos, plus a dozen of my short stories, including two about the adventures of William Walsh, which have proved popular. My regular readers are a handful of family and friends, and the blog also attracts about a hundred others a month from all over the world, and one kind donation. Thank you, whoever you are.

More importantly, the blog has helped me crystallise my own thoughts and feelings and helped me get to know many wonderful people from around the world. It won a Bloggers' Choice Award and has slowly grown in popularity. I was adding old stories and occasionally writing new ones as I started to set out my understanding of the world and my place in it. Maybe I could use my experiences to help people coming to terms with life with a disability? Maybe through my love of writing?

Social media

Social media has been key to developing my understanding of disability and the experiences of disabled people. I joined Facebook in 2007, when it was still for sharing photos of holidays or pets and catching up with old friends. Facebook enabled me to follow friends and connect with others with ataxia around the world. It is a useful network for my activism and blog. But it fed my fear of missing out. Even though I know that people post the best sides of themselves and are chasing an algorithm to show that off, I was easily convinced that everyone posting was happier than me. Better homes, kids, relationships, jobs, holidays, birthdays … just happier lives. It's the 'perfect world syndrome' – the ideal world you can never achieve. Thinking about what I was 'missing out on' was damaging for me as a person. Helen, of course, saw right through it all – she still does not use social media at all. It was useful that one of us did, but it also upset me and made feelings of jealousy, insecurity and anxiousness arise. In addition, the proportion of advertising and disagreeable socio-political posts on there has grown alarmingly. If Helen or I search for something on Google, helpful websites selling similar items in the US often pop up in my timeline for weeks afterwards.

Twitter has been a much more positive experience. I really started using it in 2018. If you choose to be honest about who you are, there are a lot of positive aspects to it. My full name is my Twitter handle; I am fully responsible for the words I use. I love the interconnectedness, the feeling of being at the centre of the world. I learned a lot of new ideas that have influenced my thinking, including some new acronyms and insults, and have made friends with people I started following on Twitter. There are so many tribes or groups, like an extended family to share your problems with. I was encouraged to see how strong the disability movement actually is, and because disabled people express their whole selves, how it overlaps and merges with other oppressed identities, the real generosity and kindness of my fellow users never ceases to remind me that the world is not all bad.

As an aside into the world of pornography ... seriously. Disabled people enjoy sex, you know! It might be me that has changed. I have found that internet pornography has become more and more distasteful, with its violence, raceplay, rape or incest fantasies, or just plain humiliation. It is chilling to think that some people think this is what sex is. Since 2019, I have subscribed to makelovenotporn, which showcases '#RealWorldSex in all its glorious, silly, beautiful, messy, reassuring humanness.' Real couples sharing videos of their most intimate moments, and actually communicating with each other. It also shares half the profits with the contributors themselves. A sense of community – this is what is missing from the world.

Twitter provides that community, but it also forces you to see yourself. Aspects of my own identity that I take for granted (White, male, heterosexual) are thrown into sharp relief against a backdrop of the decades of oppression other people have faced. I have found hearing the voices of women, people of colour, LGBTQ+, and older people, either with no disabilities or with different disabilities to mine, to be an enlightening and deeply humbling experience. This sense of community is a wonderful thing, but it has a very dark side too. I have learned many new concepts on Twitter:

- Ableism – abusing disabled people
- Ghosting – deliberately ignoring another
- Trolling – online provocation
- Dogwhistle – repeatedly using key words linked to harmful ideas
- Doxing – going through somebody's online history to find incriminating evidence
- Gaslighting – the psychological manipulation of an individual or group to question their own beliefs and their sanity.

I see that last one around us every day. With the rise of populism in the US and the UK, we are being divided and turned against each other. People in America argue with one another over abortion and gun control, while in the UK we have Brexit and culture wars, and both with a dollop of climate change and immigration. Both sides claim to be right, whilst dismissing opposing arguments as outright lies. Truth is twisted and facts perverted. We can passionately disagree with others, but some use the anonymity offered by Twitter to be rude, abusive, and unkind, or cite the term 'fake news' for any discussion they disagree with. In a war of fiercely held opinions, Twitter is the frontline. With so much outrage and anger on display, rather than open and honest debate, I wonder if such forms of social media are just a diversion that can actually stop people from taking direct action.

I get my daily news via Twitter, but have learned to treat it with great care. Since its new ownership in 2022, there is more advertising and the return of banned accounts. The whole platform has also become quite unstable. Like life, it is what you make it. Be careful who you follow and the places you go. Above all, be kind to other people and always be yourself.

I think of myself as a 'slactivst' because I'm well informed about disability, but avoid risk by staying in the background. I'm not on the frontline preaching about disability rights or chaining myself to railings (yet). The MBE has raised my profile and given me a platform, so I will get more involved.

Ableism (or how disabled people are 'cancelled')

I think of ableism as a new concept. Sadly, it is only new to me. Part of understanding disability is understanding the attitudes to disability and disabled people. 'Ableism' is discrimination against disabled people. Ableist attitudes are perpetrated by people's attitudes and expressed through the inaccessible physical environment and services we all have to live with. Ableism is a noun; something grubby, aggressive and nasty, like sexism or racism, but something that is done exclusively to disabled people. At last, ableism gives us a mechanism that shows a negative approach to disability.

As soon as I started using Twitter regularly, I quickly picked up on the strength of emotion that ableism was inflicting on other disabled people around the world. Ableism has had a tremendous impact on me. From struggling with ideas of sickness and shame, to using aids such as a wheelchair or glasses. As a wheelchair user, structural inequalities in the way we build our world and the way that most things aren't designed for me to use is the most obvious way that ableism affects me every day. This is visible to me in the narrow doorways, eye-wateringly steep ramps, flights of steps, unreachable shelves, counters and cashpoints, being left on a train, people addressing my partner instead of me, obstructed views at venues, vehicles parked on pavements, curbs designed like cliffs that presumably I am supposed to jump from to get anywhere, the rare accessible toilet filled with spare furniture, dentist chairs, public transport or taxis turning around and speeding off when they see me. Ableism plagues all disabled people in many different ways, but it always comes down to prejudice. The hardest thing for people to understand is that ableism does not *need* to exist. It is deeply rooted in society and lives and thrives in the attitudes and behaviours of *other people*.

I think there is a socially accepted hierarchy of disability. After all – I'm a White, middle-aged man in a manual wheelchair. I have a wedding ring, can move around independently and communicate well. I know I'm lucky. People who have hidden disabilities, or are Black, female or depend on a powerchair, frequently experience misogyny, racism or being assaulted.

When I was diagnosed, I had to grieve for, and come to terms with, the loss of all the things I decided I would never get to do, the person I would never get to be. I had internalised these measures of success an ableist society holds dear. I spent the next twenty years struggling to achieve those things – so I could think of myself as a 'successful' human being. This idea of 'overcoming' can be seen in the perception that our Paralympians have 'overcome their disability'. Nothing against Paralympians, I know a few and how much work they put in to accommodate an impairment in an elite sport. However, to say their example is something *all* disabled people should aspire to is very dangerous. It gives the message that disability can be overcome with hard work and positivity (or the reverse: disabled people are lazy and irredeemably negative).

When, and how, do other people develop ideas of what is normal and become terrified of being different? As a regular volunteer at my daughter's primary school, I was the only wheelchair user and one of the only men the pupils saw regularly. I would go and speak to the reception classes about disability. I would tell them quite simply that: 'My wheelchair is a tool, like a car or shoes or a bike that I use to get around.' This made perfect sense to them. I braced myself for the usual questions – 'What happened to you?' and 'How long have you been like this?' To my great delight, it quickly became clear that at 3 and 4 years old, these kids had no concept of disability, race, or gender. Perhaps that's why I enjoy working with them. My favourite question was: 'Where do you sleep?' This threw me; did they think I slept in a coffin like a vampire? They were being eminently practical; they thought that as the chair was a physical part of me, did I take it to bed with me? It is good to know we are not born afraid of, or disgusted by, disability. As we grow, we form our attitudes and behaviours from our parents, peers, and the world around us. It's called socialisation.

Unfortunately, the world around us is unfit for disabled people. I've already mentioned the structural difficulties above caused by how spaces are constructed. The workplace is similarly constructed to our disadvantage. Not just physically, but based in our value systems and our expectations of disabled people. There are institutional barriers. Disabled people are portrayed as scroungers by the mainstream media, that they don't want to work. This really isn't the case. Disabled workers (as with every minority) feel they have to work harder to push against society's dominant idea of disabled people as 'sick' and 'incapable'. The fact that we are still undervalued in the employment market proves this. According to the Office for National Statistics, in the UK in 2021, disabled workers were doing jobs that paid 13.8% less than other workers.

The situation is more that, in its current form, working does not fit with disability. It can be adapted to fit, although not very well or for very long. The problem is the idea that work must be 'productive' and even finding work is a competitive process. This idea of work disables people much more than what we simply can or can't do. It is just not practical to provide all of the support many of us would need to get to, and function in, the traditional workplace.

But there isn't just a problem with perception; it's also a question of hostile governmental practices. The Joseph Rowntree Foundation found that in 2020, half of the 14 million people living in poverty in the UK are disabled or live with a disabled person. The hostile environment continues to push disabled people and their carers into early graves. A regressive welfare system in the UK, for instance, makes it even harder to make the transition from benefits to work.

Doing anything with a disability comes with hidden costs. A government scheme called Access to Work, which supports disabled people either with an employer or a start-up business, paid for my taxis to work, adjustments to buildings, and even a new wheelchair after it broke spectacularly on the steep hill outside my office in Birmingham. Managing and submitting receipts was OK when I got used to doing it. Ten years after I used it, the Access to Work Scheme still exists, as does the disabled students allowance I claimed when I was a student; although invaluable to my quality of work life (making work possible), both have been heavily cut and capped. In August 2020, the DWP claimed that it would be extending this scheme to support disabled workers through the global pandemic. What is work without meaning? A YouGov poll in 2020 found that a quarter of British workers found their jobs lack meaning. I have found a lot of satisfaction through non-paid work. However, not everyone is in the same position as I am to afford to do this. Volunteering provides meaning, but also removes the financial reward.

A new hope

We cannot rely on a vague hope that things will change, we need to make that change happen.

I Googled 'hope' and found thousands of quotes. All very profound, said by mostly inspirational people, mostly men, and against a picture of a sunset or a dove or a green shoot in a desert. This included quotes from heroes of mine who are no longer with us: John Lennon, Martin Luther King Jr., Jim Henson, David Bowie, Robin Williams, Malcolm X, Christopher Reeve and Norman Wisdom. They all talked about what hope meant to them; are dead men the only people who can give us hope?

Following my diagnosis, and spurred on by the desperate hope of my parents, I tried everything; I had a healing crystal dangled and healing words chanted over me. I wasn't actually ill, so couldn't really tell if I had been cured or not. I knew my condition was incurable, an inescapable death sentence, but – deep down – the Catholic schoolboy in me believed that somehow a miracle might happen. I now know that while my future would probably be shaped by scientific progress, how I live with my disability each day is my responsibility. I try to live in the moment, where hoping for a cure is fanciful, dangerous, and bogus.

Then, in October 2019, I had to reassess my relationship with hope and my whole identity after Reata, a global pharmaceutical company, announced promising results on a study of patients with my condition. Initial results from a 48-week trial of the drug Omaveloxolone (Omav) showed that it improves mitochondrial function and can slow the progression of Friedreich's ataxia. It was fast-tracked by the Food and Drug Administration (FDA) in America and was predicted to be available in the US from summer 2023. Reata are hoping to bring it to the European market in 2024. How much is a miracle cure worth? How much can hope be sold for? In this instance, subject to cruel market forces, it is expected to cost $300,000 per year. This puts it beyond the reach of those without medical insurance and will generate immense debt and disappointment within our community. What is the point of offering hope and keeping it out of reach?

At least hope is out there, alongside real movement towards a treatment or cure. I have never allowed myself to dream what my life could have been like or would be like now if there was one. It raises troublesome thoughts. Although in my dreams, I am never in a wheelchair. I'm forever at the time when I could not walk very far or well. I often dream about finding a toilet, only to find it unusable in some way. For the first time, I can playfully wonder out loud what it would be like to learn to walk again and, here's the downside, eventually have to go back to work in my fifties.

I have learned that I don't need a cure to make me complete or happy. Mourning the loss disability brings with it is important, but only so you can let the past go and move forwards. The real value in life is the things we do in the present. Would a miracle cure mean that the heroic struggle that has made me who I am, everything I have worked so hard to do, all been for nothing? What if, after being cured, I got hit by a bus or was diagnosed with cancer? Would I have wasted all my time hoping for a cure? Consciously letting go of false hope has helped me form my own identity and live a successful life in the present, instead of chasing an unclear future. I know medication wouldn't make me 'whole' again, for I already am a whole person, but I would be delighted if my condition could be stabilised – even at this more advanced stage.

Hope is similar to wishful thinking. It can sustain our physical bodies, but it is fleeting and unstable. The problem with hope is that it can reassure us that we are just spectators, that we don't need to take matters into our own hands. Holocaust survivor, wounded healer and psychologist Viktor Frankl witnessed how deaths increased inexplicably in Auschwitz just after Christmas. He believed that in the New Year, as the hope his fellow inmates had that they would be home by that Christmas had gone, they started to give up on life. A survivor of four camps, he observed (Frankl, 2004) that it wasn't necessarily the physically fit who survived longest, but those who used their hope to develop a sense of meaning and purpose from their suffering.

I believe the best way to develop precious hope is to use careful optimism to target meaning and purpose. Frankl calls this 'practical optimism'. In an interview in 2019, Mike Oliver, pioneer of the social model of disability, said, 'It (equality) was about having an optimistic view of what disabled people could achieve if many of the barriers they faced were removed.'

Michael J Fox shows us how to blend optimism with gratitude. After his diagnosis with Parkinson's, he describes his relationship with disability (Fox, 2020). What has really been key to maintaining his optimism is the confidence gained from his natural understanding of the social model of disability. The kind of insight you develop from years of living with a disability and being around clever people who do too. He is an optimist. He is not living for a cure, but because life has meaning for him. His impairment is a challenge, but his Parkinson's does not define him. He knows that those who love him see what he can do, rather than what he can't; he sees a wheelchair as a tool to make his life easier; and he retired from acting with reason and good grace, explaining that acting doesn't owe him anything. He is grateful for the amazing experiences and opportunities acting gave, and accepts it cannot give him any more. I like how he does this; it's not that he can't do the acting, it's that acting no longer works for him. It may have taken 18 years, but he is immune to the negativity of 'other people.'

This turning of hope into practical optimism is the aim of the 'All About Ataxia' workshops. Most attendees come along with little or no hope left. It has been knocked out of them. By sharing our stories and giving an overall positive message, we show how they can influence the progression of their ataxia themselves. It's those words again, 'You gotta buy a ticket!' Life doesn't stop with a diagnosis but it is the beginning of a new, distinct struggle. By helping people take more control of their health and live a more comfortable life, we try to plant a seed of optimism.

We must remember that for many disabled people, a cure is not possible. What we should hope for, and all work toward, is equity in a just and compassionate society. We can only make this happen if we understand ourselves.

George Harrison

Following a series of coincidental mentions, my attention was drawn to George Harrison. He had always been in the background as the 'quiet Beatle', but I was now seeing him as a gifted artist in his own right – someone I had overlooked. He was clearly an exceptional person, beloved of so many and had searched for his own identity; I was determined to learn more about him. I went deeper, convinced that he had a message for me!

I began with the closest thing there is to an autobiography; *I, Me, Mine* (Harrison G. , 2017) is a collection of autobiographical writings, photographs, and original song lyrics with brief recollections shared for each. Clearly written for a small circle of friends, this book was first released as a limited edition of 2,000 hand-bound and signed copies in 1980. After his death, it was extended and re-published in 2002 and again in 2017. To give the book an extra dimension, I listened to each of the 141 songs as I read.

George's recollections of his early years have a raw, simplistic, underdeveloped feel to them, quite matter-of-fact. Often, he will introduce a theme or an idea, explain it, then close it down by simply saying, 'Well, that's how it was'. George is quick to set out early on that he does not see any value in talking about himself and does not give his time as a Beatle any special emphasis. Similarly, the fascinating stories about his path to spirituality, lifelong legal battles for privacy, how he fought an epic guitar dual with Eric Clapton, broke up Ringo Starr's marriage or mortgaged his home to finance the Monty Python film *Life of Brian* are left untold. This could point to a difficult or obtuse character, but it is in his handwritten lyrics and the short paragraphs he provides for many of his songs that you really begin to get a sense of him. Not that he makes it easy.

I think that is the point of *I, Me, Mine*. Far from a sense of modesty or a lack of ability to express his feelings, George was content to leave those stories for others to tell – he just happened to be there. He was aware that his ego was part of a larger consciousness and he didn't see any point in inflating it. A hint is in the title of the book. 'I Me Mine' is a song about the ego and its part of a greater consciousness. After all, 'The Lord doesn't manifest through ego,' George says.

John Lennon fell into this trap. He was not impressed when he received his copy as he felt it didn't give him any credit as one of George's influences. Just four days after John Lennon's murder, George rewrote 'All Those Years Ago' and dedicated it to his friend: 'I always looked up to you' and 'You were the one who imagined it all, all those years ago.' Now Lennon was part of a bigger consciousness, now was the moment to recognise his contribution. For me, that sums up how George was.

Spirituality was important to George. His early experiences with LSD altered his perception of reality, and himself, and prompted a spiritual journey which lasted for the rest of his life. For him, God is more a concept of enlightenment found through meditation, and beliefs in karma and reincarnation, than the judgemental, vengeful, and controlling God of Western tradition. His path to enlightenment seems to have been through the teachings of Buddha and the Hindu religion. If Zen can only be found in the obliteration of the self, this suited the ex-Beatle just fine. Rather than the descending path (the appreciation of community, nature, earth, life, other people, and looking outward), George was more interested in the ascending path to enlightenment. This focuses on the individual and their personal relationship with God. Although on this path, he did not feel the need to cut his hair or give up alcohol. As an atheist, I was disappointed that I would not be able to follow his path, but was heartened to learn that there is a strong tradition of atheism in Hinduism.

George's widow, Olivia, recently published a moving tribute (Harrison, 2022) of 20 poems, one for each year since he died. The love she feels for him is still with her. I wrote to their son, Dhani, a couple of years younger than me, and suggested we meet up.

Helen did say it would be difficult not to come across as creepy (I never had a reply).

George wrote beautiful songs about peace, spoke out about inequality, touched so many people, and was completely surrounded by love. He was a complex person, and his was a difficult and unusual journey. Most of all, I admire his rejection of ego and the deep love he inspired in others. This was the wisdom I was seeking, someone telling me to let go of everything beyond my control and have faith in the universe.

I, ME, MINE

The profound changes that people around me were going through convinced me that my own self-reflection was overdue. That I look at myself deeply and disconnect my ego from my condition. We cannot ignore the physical aspects of our impairments as we age. After all, we can do most things, just differently. There are ways to keep doing what you love and keep finding meaning in your life. We all experience pain and fatigue in different ways. Let's be understanding, accepting, and open about this. If we don't understand our own bodies, society has already disabled us.

People often say that they are impressed because I 'don't complain much.' This is a backhanded compliment at best. I don't talk about my disability because that would be seen as complaining and I would feel embarrassed and ashamed. After all, nobody wants to hear how you really are. To avoid judgement, disabled people have to keep quiet about their health. An ableist society puts us under great pressure to show grit, steel, and courage instead.

I've talked about how I lived in denial of my condition until I retired, but I don't think I embraced it properly until a friend presented a video about her life with ataxia at our virtual conference in 2020. As she spoke openly about her care needs, I began to think 'Whoa, this is way too much information.' It made me consider the extent of my efforts to cover up my disability, and why I was doing it. It also made me appreciate the privileged position I enjoy as a visibly disabled, middle-aged, middle-class, heterosexual, White man. So, thanks to Emma, a fellow volunteer with Ataxia UK during the first lockdown in 2020, here is a full and frank description of how my disability affects my life.

My energy is limited and I feel tired all the time. My wrists, elbows and shoulders ache from the strain of nearly thirty years of propelling myself in a wheelchair. My scoliosis (curvature of the spine) makes sitting or lying down uncomfortable, so my lower back aches from sitting in a wheelchair. Sometimes I feel like my body is slowly curling into itself. Poor circulation means my hands and feet (possibly exasperated by Raynaud's syndrome) are painfully cold through winter. In the summer, they swell up and sweat soaks my back from sitting in a wheelchair all day. My transfers are generally poor and require a lot of concentration. I fall a few times a year – thankfully not very far. If we go out in the car, Helen folds my chair and lifts it into the back of the car. I am grateful to her for enabling much of my independence.

I have no reactions to speak of but jump out of my skin and have an adrenaline-fuelled fight-or-flight reaction to loud and sudden noises. I have tinnitus, a high frequency background noise, and hearing loss known as auditory neuropathy. I can still hear sound clearly, I just cannot separate the frequencies of different sounds. I only hear the loudest one. For example, in a noisy restaurant, I cannot hear a person next to me talking, all I can hear is the background noise. This kind of hearing loss is often linked to cognitively impaired perception of speech. I have always been frustrated at my inability to follow what people who have difficulties with speech are saying and have always found it difficult to focus on details and remember names.

Although I have my toenails cut by a podiatrist and need some help getting dressed, I can manage all my own personal care. My eyesight is stable, but is now at the very limits of what corrective lenses can do. I need reading glasses, but suspect that is an age-related problem. Difficulty focusing (nystagmus) makes watching quick movement difficult. My speech is slower and slightly slurred and I can manage to write a signature or single words (like death) IN CAPITAL LETTERS that soon become unreadable, but nothing more.

My grip is weak and I cannot manage full pint glasses anymore. As I eat one-handed, I use my other arm to keep myself upright and find cutting food difficult. I prefer foods you can eat with a fork or just hold in your hand. I need to concentrate on swallowing liquid or I'll choke. Triggered by coughing or a shock, my involuntary leg spasms make for the most interesting disruptions. I remember seeing a play in Stratford, I had extended my legs so my feet were under the chairs of the elderly couple in front. A gunshot in the auditorium (part of the action) shocked me into bringing my feet up sharply into the bottom of their seats. You should have seen them jump and look round, trying to work out if they were the only members of the audience with special vibrating seats! I returned their looks of disbelief and looked around too, sharing in their concern.

I have difficulties with urgency when toileting and need to be careful what I eat and make sure I drink enough water. Fatigue and poor mobility coupled with middle age and two children make sexual fulfilment much more of a challenge. I recently stopped eating gluten and drinking coffee and am pleased with the difference it has made (not in the bedroom, sorry to disappoint!). My middle-aged body just cannot do all the things it used to, and certainly not as quickly. Instead of being bitter about the things I can't do, I need to recognise them and appreciate the things I can do.

I use a speech-to-text programme to help me

write for sustained periods. I listen to music and audiobooks, watch TV and film, play on my PlayStation, and can use computers and phone apps adequately. I get out and about on my trike and I exercise with my THERA-trainer for about an hour every day. This helps with my digestion and cardio. I sleep fitfully.

I never understood what depression and anxiety were, but I know they have always been with me. As a child of the '80s, there were plenty of things to worry about: nuclear war, punk rockers, my parents divorcing or a Dalek invasion. Now our children can add a pandemic, zombies, climate change, the far right, global war and conspiracy theories to that list. Today, I feel depression's pull when I am at my lowest, perhaps after a fall, short of sleep or fighting off illness. I recognise that those first 25 years after my diagnosis were when I had the energy to be much more active, but I don't consider the time I spent 'chasing normal' to be wasted. I self-manage my own health as I feel abandoned by the healthcare system. As George Harrison observed, 'We spend too much effort treating illness, not keeping people well.' This has saved me hours of travelling, constantly having to explain my condition, and living with the side effects of the many drugs I would be prescribed to mitigate my symptoms. I'm glad I have done this for as long as I could, but I feel I may have missed out on important support when I needed it, especially now when my needs are more complex.

Once I had taken the time to 'see myself' as things

were, it was well overdue that I recognised 'my inner child' (my ego) and take his grubby hands off the steering wheel of my life. The bravery, vulnerability and redemption of John Lennon, the powerful optimism of Michael J. Fox, the self-discovery of Chris McCandless, the rejection of ego of George Harrison were key elements of the person I wanted to be more like.

How would I describe my inner child? His childhood was happy, but he is a privileged, golden child. He struggles with low self-esteem and being assertive. The promise of a chronic disability, with hardly any physical signs – and those that did would creep up so slowly that he would not be aware of them – locked him into a hopeless existence. He was cast into the bleakest nihilism when he was 15. Preoccupied with appearances, he has always craved attention and spends too much time thinking about or seeking it. He is driven by it: to be wanted. It is a powerful addiction he cannot control. He overthinks, becomes jealous, resentful, and sulky if he does not get enough. He carries with him a very unfair idea of relationships, based in the traditional gender roles he saw all around him as a child. He has a short temper and does not deal with criticism well. I wouldn't say he is dysfunctional, just very difficult to manage sometimes.

I see him at work in my marriage. Like everyone's, mine has had its rough patches. As we have grown older, the emotional, expressive side of our relationship has changed, but not disappeared completely. Sometimes, my feelings of low self-esteem bubble up and I feel threatened and deeply jealous, and like a burden, an inconvenience. In these moments, I am afraid that our marriage has become a trap. That Helen has checked out and is waiting for me to die so she can be free at last. Honestly, I wouldn't blame her.

My disability has not helped. It has increased my dependency on others and my frustration with myself has had an impact on my self-esteem. I realised that I had caused or made these problems feel much worse than they were and that I was in control of those thoughts. The paranoia, insecurity, blaming others, the unrealistic expectations, sulking, lashing out; I didn't want that anymore.

Then, overthinking as usual, I wondered if *not* listening to my inner child was such a good idea. After all, he was very good at denial, and had served me well in that department over the years. I realised that rather than ignore parts that we don't like, it is important to recognise those parts of ourselves and choose to act differently. I want to be more aware of myself and other people. I have taken a break from Facebook to see if that would help ground my expectations. It has, but the root of the problem goes much deeper. I have a problem with managing negative thoughts. I construct situations in my mind and feed off the negative emotion that I have created, as if investing oneself too much into a film. That is a part of me I have to recognise, understand, and challenge.

I know that living in the present is more than just denying the future – the mind has to be trained to stick to it. I have been able to disconnect from my conscious self, but need to do some work and study meditation properly. But letting go and trusting in the universe, higher power, or God – as George Harrison did? That is advanced. Maybe that could be something for me to aspire to – the nirvana you never quite reach because you are not humble enough.

Communal drumming

I had tasted the spiritual sense of belonging through sharing music in a crowd, either at football matches or at concerts. By chance, I found that music was the key I needed to unlock my own subconscious. Bella won a family ticket to a local music festival and I went along with my trike. In a family-friendly layout, there were several big top tents. One had a few people in it, sitting cross-legged and playing drums. I have always struggled when trying to meditate as part of a group. I find that the noise of my everyday thoughts is too difficult to silence and I just cannot relax enough. I always end up sitting and looking enviously at others in the group enjoying their own meditative state. At the centre of this tent, one person was standing up and setting the rhythm for everyone. *Just a random bunch of hippies*, I thought dismissively. Yes, I'm guilty of forming quick initial impressions too! The floor was littered with drums of all different shapes and sizes, so that everyone could join in. Why not? I liked the inclusive nature of this. Hovering around the edge of the group, I selected a big black pair of drums and began to find the rhythm. Slowly we were joined by others and the rhythm got more intense. I began by playing within the rhythm; it tethered me to the sound and soon I was playing complex counter rhythms alongside. My mind had emptied and I really started to enjoy feeling part of this collective. Being a part of the rhythm was like being carried along in a river. Afterwards, I realised it had finally happened, I had at last been able to let go of my thoughts in a group. In fact, the group were a very important part of it. The magic of community.

How to live with a disability

We need to understand disability better and how it affects how we are seen and how we see ourselves. The problems faced by disabled people are intertwined with the problems of our society. We must take a global perspective to recognise and promote human rights and the intersectionality between the billions of us around the world. Failure to do this has terrible consequences for *all* groups seeking equality. As Percy Bysshe Shelley says in his poem, *The Masque of Anarchy*, 'We are many, they are few.'

There is always someone who enjoys telling you

what is wrong. I look for people who tell you what needs to change and how to make it happen. So, here it is.

Me, I'm still learning. Here are some of the things I think helped me and will help anyone with a disability, especially those new to life with a disability, get the most from life. Friends and family must give the support we need to do this. The way we go about this has changed forever with the pandemic, but they are necessary and, above all, possible.

1. Educate yourself: Understand disability and your rights

Disabled people are already in a terrible position. We find our rights significantly weakened because we are seen as sick, burdensome and tragic victims. At the same time, we are pressurised to get better, be inspirational superachievers, and prove how sick we are. The following resources will help you understand where these conflicting messages come from, how they are playing out right now and how disabled people are organising for change:

- *Disability: The Basics* by Tom Shakespeare (Routeledge, 2017). This book explains disability, but does so by looking at the lived experience of disabled people all around the world and through history.
- Disability News Service: https://www.

disabilitynewsservice.com The country's only news agency specialising in disability issues.
- Disability Rights UK: https://www.disabilityrightsuk.org. Campaigning organisation run by and for disabled people.

If we can understand how disability works in our society – who the gatekeepers are and the barriers we will face; the shame we are made to feel and why other people treat us so poorly – we will be able to make the best use of our limited energy to be ourselves.

An important part of this understanding is that we reject the labels that other people place on disabled people. Don't accept sympathy for being disabled. Be proud.

2. Be assertive, be resilient

Unfair and exhausting as it is, you and/or someone close to you will have to become your advocate. We are taught to respect authority, never to question it. A lot of people just accept what they are told. Don't. You have to become a fighter, yet choose your fights carefully. You deserve to be listened to; your lived experience is just as important as anyone else's. Tell professionals what you need them to do for you, and question what you are told. A 'sick' person has little or no privacy and most people will behave like that toward you. They may ask personal questions that they have no right to ask, or give 'help' without offering it first. No matter how well intentioned they may be, other people need to learn to respect disabled people. We need to call out ableism whenever we see it.

Keep trying. Being told 'no' can have different meanings, it never means 'stop trying.'

3. Be present, be optimistic

Easier said than done. We may not be able to overcome our impairments, but we can live fulfilling lives *with* them. Disability is a constant in our lives so try to focus on the moment. Live in the present, do not live in denial, guard your limited energies to manage living day-to-day. Pick your fights ,as being angry all the time is a waste of your precious energy and makes life difficult for those around you. Small, daily accomplishments are important to celebrate.

Hope is a cycle. Even If you have none, you can generate some by finding purpose and meaning in your life. By embracing optimism and gratitude, we can influence the things we can change and let go of those we can't. It isn't possible to avoid depression every day, but on our good days we can pass a little hope to others.

Living with a progressive condition is another reason for living in the moment. As Michael J Fox says in his recent documentary (Guggenheim, 2023), 'This condition is bigger than us, it will win.

We'll get one chance to hit back and hurt it.' You can make a difference, but you have a rapidly closing window of opportunity in which to do it. In life, good things only happen if we foster the opportunity for them to occur, through hard work and resilience.

4. Become an expert, not a victim

Even though a condition may be incurable, an entire range of therapies, aids and activities can significantly improve your physical health and mental wellbeing.

A doctor may have trained for ten years or longer, but doesn't have the lived experience you have. Sometimes, medical professionals adopt an entitled, paternalist approach to your health and usually only focus on a cure. There are very few who have a holistic view of disability. Maybe these individuals have experience of disability themselves, but they are few and far between.

From my experience and from speaking to a lot of people with ataxia, you should not expect any of the professionals you come into contact with to automatically have a good understanding of your condition. Your relationship with your medical professionals is a long-term one, their support can be invaluable and worth working on. You can take the responsibility for your own wellbeing, but be prepared to educate the medical professionals you meet, then they will be better able to help you.

5. Believe in yourself and leave people who don't behind

Other people generally have very low or no expectations of what disabled people can do. For every person who will encourage you, there are ten who will tell you exactly why you shouldn't or can't. You know who these people are. Your energy is limited and precious, you cannot waste it on people who don't deserve it. Wish them well and leave them behind. Always believe in yourself. Making new friends is easier; you now have something in common with most people: you've been pushed to the edge of society. Surround yourself with people who truly believe in you. The kind of people that will support you as you decide what you want to do and can achieve. The kind of people that will tell you what we all need to hear in our darkest moments: you are not alone, you are loved, you are wonderful, and you are enough. Sharing life with these people is much more joyous and meaningful than doing it on your own. A quick and easy way of finding empathy and comfort is through having contact with people in your patient group. Meeting people in situations like yours is great, but remember that your experience is unique to you and be aware that there are plenty of people with your condition that will never share your approach to life.

But what can **we** do?

In the '90s, there was a strong disability movement. Protesters used direct action to protest against the awful treatment they endured through their lack of rights. The Disability Discrimination Act came into force in 1995 and those legal protections were enshrined in the Equality Act 2010. Even though the prospect of winning a court case against an employer or service provider is beyond the means of most disabled people, we had the medical and social models of disability to explain that disability is imposed on us by other people and the environment we live in.

Those pioneers are gone, but that hope was captured in the opening ceremony of the 2012 Olympic Games. Our national story laid out, with the evils of our world vanquished by NHS doctors and nurses. I went to the 2012 Paralympic Games and greatly enjoyed the sense of inclusion that I found there. It was the first and only time I felt truly welcome in London. It is chilling to think of how far we have fallen since. I hope future generations will change these terrible attitudes and environments once and for all.

We are living in dark times at the moment. I just don't think it is safe for disabled people to be visible. At present, mask-wearing in public places and regular testing are not required, and vaccinations are not available for all. The air in our schools, public buildings, and workplaces is not filtered. The safety nets of our NHS and social care systems have been run down and allowed to collapse. Out-of-control capitalism has drained all the good from our communities and pushed disabled people and many others into poverty. There are an estimated 65 million people globally with long Covid, with 1 in 10 having to stop working. This is projected to rise to 200 million in ten years. Many disabled people have been left with no option but to continue isolating.

We need to develop the social model of disability to recognise and address the experiences of, and barriers against, people with all impairments. Our mental health and the very real pain and fatigue we all feel. Our best hope for accomplishing this is through a strong network of Disabled People's Organisations (DPOs). Groups run by and for disabled people who are highly valued and qualified to supervise national policy. This is opposite to the current government's direction of travel. So, we educate ourselves and protest. While we still can.

We have hope things will get better, but we need to approach this hope with practical optimism. Our voices still need to be heard and our communities need to grow. We can still set an example for others. It is possible to volunteer, fundraise, raise awareness, and socialise online. Using blogs and social media, we can still make a difference and connect to the things we love.

But we also need to look beyond our own

communities and identify the problems we share with others. The mess we are in is not purely a disability problem. For a start, we need to reverse the cuts and closures we have all endured through the last 14 years of austerity. We need to begin to reverse privatisation, return our utilities to public ownership (Anna Coote, 2020), close tax loopholes, and overhaul our toxic political system – to repeal the draconian legislation passed during these times. I believe that we need to rejoin the EU, and invest heavily in education, transport, housing, social and health care, and renewable energy. We need to regulate our media and its ownership. Under the Higher Education (Freedom of Speech) Act of 2023, Universities are now required to bring 'balance' to their debates, which results in universities giving a platform to groups with no expertise and provably untrue and violent rhetoric.

Like the Black Panthers who knew the importance of supporting their communities, we need to develop an intersectional approach to discrimination. Where all oppressed groups can stand together against poverty. In the UK, 2.1 million people shouldn't be using foodbanks.

Undoing all the mistakes of 14 years of austerity would bring us back to the point where disabled people were able to flourish, as I did. I think you can guess I am about to say that it would only be the start. In our capitalist society, disabled people are judged purely by our economic value. We need to see the greatest redistribution of wealth ever – a Universal Basic Income (UBI) (Standing, 2017). This is a fixed payment with no means test and no requirement to work, for all. Such payments would finally acknowledge the important work of caregivers and volunteers.

This would stabilize job, social care and housing markets, end unpaid care, low-paid or zero-hour contract work and lift millions out of poverty in one stroke. It would provide the opportunity to replace the unpopular and costly Universal Income program with a cheaper, more efficient system that treats people with dignity. More importantly, it would enable people to find greater meaning in life by pursuing education, exploring their creativity or entrepreneurism.

Unaffordable? Much of this money would find its way back to the exchequer anyway. The current government clearly does not understand basic economics. It is a myth that governments have strict budgets to balance, just look at the UK's spiralling national deficit. Self-imposed public spending constraints (austerity) leave any government with little to no money for tax cuts or investments. The resulting streamlining our benefits system, scaling back spending on our military, and the aggressive recovery of unpaid taxes would easily cover this.

Unpopular? Certainly. 'Giving' people a basic wage with no expectation to work would be unacceptable for many. It is a very forward-thinking idea, but there are a couple of trials. The Basic Income for Care Leavers in Wales pilot targets those leaving care who are turning 18 between 1 July 2022 and 30 June 2023. Two places in England have been selected for micro pilot schemes: central Jarrow, in north-east England, and East Finchley, in north London. Each provides a monthly payment of £1,600 (£1,280, after-tax). Some recent studies (McMaster University, 2020) from Canada show positive effects of UBI.

These trials are limited and run alongside capitalism, instead of replacing it. UBI is vulnerable to corporate price-gouging:, we need to go much further and do it much faster. There is something very wrong with our society when a quarter of it is languishing in poverty. A UBI needs to be just that: universal. We need to turn away from the values which only see people in terms of productivity, sets the cost of treatments beyond the means of all but a few, and has allowed us to ravage our planet: capitalism and the relentless pursuit of profit. Extending the UBI to all would emancipate people from money forever. People would be free to use their time in meaningful ways. A very utopian idea perhaps, but something fundamental like this needs to happen if we are to survive.

We just haven't learned. I agree with John Higgs (Higgs, 2019) that it won't be us, but future generations who will make real change. They simply won't accept our fatalist view of the future and will make change happen. Perhaps they'll use radical ideas that exist now but that we've been unable to implement like a UBI or leaving half the globe to nature. It is not too late to undo some of the damage.

THE TAKEAWAY

Is disability other people? Yes.

I argue that disability is the norm; it is something we share with one billion or 15% of people around the world. We all have impairments of some kind, they can arrive at any time and get better, worse or leave us all together. Their likelihood increases with repeated Covid infections or as we get older. Even those who claim to be 'normal' know they are all just one banana skin away from being disabled themselves.

Despite our numbers, disabled people, amongst a great many others who are different, are pushed to the edges. *Other people* carry the attitudes that leads to the ableism that really disables us. They are afraid of anything different. It's understandable. Our brains aren't designed, via our limited experience, to recognise our own part in problems. Blaming someone else for your problems is much more convenient. From speeding, to climate change, immigration and public health. Unfortunately, the society we live in aggressively disables many of us and we must fight with all our strength, our resilience, our determination, and a lot of luck. If we don't, we could be part of the problem too.

There is a chronic lack of understanding of disability in general. It is in the embarrassed whispers; it is in the terrible assumptions and judgements that people make. It is in the way we are constantly dismissed and devalued. When I was diagnosed, I set my focus on achieving all the things I *thought* I should achieve: going to university, having a family, a home, a career, and learning to drive. I just needed motivation and a strong work ethic to accompany my own sense of specialness. I became part of the problem and spent the best years of my life chasing these things, not just because I was in denial, but because I was following my own internalised ableism, listening to *other people*. That choice was physically and emotionally draining but I don't regret it. I am grateful for the great love, skills, experience, and the modest financial stability it gave me. Operating within an increasingly capitalist society, that stability enabled my adventure in volunteering. With today's eye-watering debt and government cuts to support, I just cannot see how my journey can be followed by young disabled people.

We don't have to be pushed around like this. If

our challenges make us who we are, we are set apart by how we face them. But we cannot even begin to do that without the right support. This is where this concept of *other people* is problematic. Other people represent the best of us too. Fortunately, many of those people are out there too, already at the edge of society with us. I work hard as a volunteer to kindle that magic that comes when a community works together. I found it to be much more fulfilling than conventional working. I'm especially proud of my work with Ataxia UK, OurBus Bartons, Save Our Fox and getting to know some special people along the way. It is only with the support and love of those *other people* that disabled people can do great things.

The most important thing I learned is that 'you gotta buy a ticket.' I had weekly numbers for the National Lottery, for many years. I think the most I ever won was £30. I stopped those payments recently when I realised that the only ticket you need in life is yourself. Therefore, to make sure we're not part of the problem, we have to act. I've learned that we can't just rely on a vague hope to change things, we need to change the way disabled people are seen by other people, but, more importantly, we need to change how we see ourselves. Whether it's in our lives and our own situations, such as within our local community, or changing the way disability is understood in society, we need to take part. The moments in my life when I felt like I won the lottery were times when I took control. Some examples are meeting Helen, becoming a father and being awarded an MBE. So that worked out pretty well!

The pandemic, especially the lockdowns, presented me with the time to reflect on the world around me and my own life. It also changed volunteering for me, but didn't stop me finding fulfilment in it.

Volunteering, although it has never put a scrap of gold or silver in my pocket, has showed me that meaning and fulfilment, new friends and new experiences are out there for the taking. You just have to buy a ticket. Death is a useful reminder that we need to be present and to always live in the moment.

I was very ill with Covid at the end of 2022. As I was too poorly to look after myself, Helen worked with the Covid-at-Home team to keep me out of hospital. I spent twelve days in bed, too weak to move. It dramatically increased the progression of my ataxia, broke my resolve, and left me with precious little energy. My recovery has been imperceptibly slow, with constant fatigue, overwhelm, and depression. My sensitivity to light and sound are now dramatically heightened. With Covid running rampant through our environment and each reinfection increasing the chance of death, I feel abandoned once again and am reluctant to take the additional risk of going out at the moment. By not taking steps to limit the effects of the pandemic, other people have pushed me to the edge of society once again. We know that is where we find others struggling for their rights, and long-

Covid means our numbers are growing. It is from there that we need to build our networks and make change happen.

It is not just *other* people we need to change. We also need to abandon out-of-control capitalism. It is an economic system that will never value disabled people and has almost destroyed our planet.

On rare occasions, I am almost grateful for my disability, but my relationship with it is a complex one. On bad days, my condition becomes my personal nemesis, a shadowy supervillain who has gleefully taken everything from me and knows it – laughing hysterically from just beyond my reach. Disability has changed my life and I have had to make peace with it. It has helped me find the strength I need to carry on fighting to follow my dreams. It has taught me that only you can determine the quality of your own life and the importance of having the right support. My condition, and the *right* people, helped me overcome myself and briefly, for a beautiful moment, feel like a superman. Volunteering gave me the tools I needed to become a superhero. Now, as a 'wounded healer', I am slowing down, looking back, getting my 'wisdom' on paper for anyone struggling with strange, new powers of their own.

Disabled people know what it is like to be outsiders who have to begin again from nothing and fight against pain, fatigue and *other people* every day. Because of this, we are all superheroes.

ACKNOWLEDGEMENTS

I would like to express my sincere gratitude to the people who accompanied me in my journey, the people who influenced, counselled and inspired me. They helped me recognise and achieve my potential. I simply wouldn't have got here without them. Special thanks to Valeryia Steadman, whose beautiful cover art perfectly captured my superhero moment; Dr Emma Parfitt, whose expert editing and proofreading brought much needed coherence and sense-checking to this story; and to the team at Troubador for their epic support and great patience.

BIBLIOGRAPHY

Anna Coote, A. P. (2020). *The Case for Universal Basic Services.* Polity.

British Skydiving. (2023, February). Retrieved from https://britishskydiving.org/how-safe/#:~:text=The%20all%2D time%20tandem%20fatality,carries%20the%20lowest%20 risk%20profile.

Cippola, C. (2011). *The Basic Laws of Human Stupidity.* Il Mulino.

Clifford, E. (2020). *The War on Disabled People: Capitalism, Welfare and the Making of a Human Catastrophe.* Zed Books.

Coleman, R. (1995). *John Lennon – The Definitive Biography.* Pan Books.

Colin in Black and White (TV mini series) (2021). [Motion Picture].

Commission on Race and Ethnic Disparities. (2021). *The report of the Commission on Race and Ethnic Disparities.*

Cross, C. R. (2002). *Heavier Than Heaven: The Biography of Kurt Cobain.* Sseptre.

Dickens, C. (2022). *A Christmas Carol: The Original Classic Story.*

Ende, M. (1988). *The Neverending Story.* Penguin.

English, O. (2022). *Fake History: Ten Great Lies and How They Shaped the World.* Audible Studios.

English, O. (2023). *Fake Heroes: Ten False Icons and How They Altered the Course of History.* Welbeck.

Fox, M. J. (2003). *Lucky Man: A Memoir.* Ebury Press.
Fox, M. J. (2020). *No Time Like the Future: An Optimist Considers His Mortality.* Headlline Publishing Group.
Frankl, V. E. (2004). *Man's Search for Meaning.* Blackstone Audio Inc.
Gaiman, N. (2020). *The Sandman.* Audible Originals. Retrieved from The Sandman.
Guggenheim, D. (Director). (2023). *Still: A Michael J Fox Film* [Motion Picture].
Haley, A. (1987). *The Autobiography of Malcolm X: As Told to Alex Haley.* Doubleday.
Harrison, G. (2017). *I, Me, Mine.* Genesis Publications.
Harrison, O. (2022). *Came the Lightning: Twenty Poems for George.* Genesis Publications.
Harvey, D. (2005). *A Brief History of Neoliberalism.* Oxford University Press.
Hatfield, H. W. (2013). *The Superhero Reader.* University Press of Mississippi.
Higgs, J. (2019). *The Future Starts Here: An Optimistic Guide to What Comes Next.* Orion Publishing Group.
Higgs, J. (2022). *Love and Let Die: Bond, The Beatles and the British Pyshe.* Weidenfeld & Nicolson.
Krakauer, J. (2011). *Into the Wild.* Pan.
Masefield, J. (1984). *The Box of Delights.* Lions.
McMaster University. (2020, March). *Southern Ontario's Basic Income Experience.* Retrieved from https://labourstudies.socsci.mcmaster.ca/documents/southern-ontarios-basic-income-experience.pdf
Morris, T. (2005). *Superheroes and Philosophy: Truth, Justice, and the Socratic Way (Popular Culture and Philosophy).* Open Court.
Newnham, J. L. (Director). (2020). *Crip Camp* [Motion Picture].
Obama, B. (2020). *A Promised Land.* Random House.
Office for National Statistics. (2020, June) Retrieved from https://www.ons.gov.uk/people populationand community/wellbeing/articles/coronavirusandanxietygreatbritain/3april2020to10may2020/pdf

Office for National Statistics. (2020). *Coronavirus (COVID-19) related deaths by disability status, England and Wales: 2 March to 14 July 2020.*

Pratchett, T. (1992). *Small Gods.* Gollancz.

Refuge. (2020). Retrieved from https://refuge.org.uk/news/25-increase-in-calls-to-national-domestic-abuse- helpline-since-lockdown-measures-began/#:~:text=Refuge%2C%20the%20UK's%20largest%20domestic,t%20reason%20for%20abusive%20behaviour.

Retrieved from Disability Rights Commission. (2020, January) https://www.disabilityrightsuk.org/news/2020/january/over-100000-dla-claimants-lose-motability-vehicles-after-pip-reassessment

Sanghera, S. (2021). *Empireland: How Imperialism Has Shaped Modern Britain.* Viking.

Satre, J. P. (2013). *No Exit.* Samuel French inc.

Scope. (2020, May). Retrieved from https://www.scope.org.uk/campaigns/disabled-people-and-coronavirus/the-disability-report/

Shakespeare, T. (2017). *Disability: The Basics.* Routledge.

Standing, G. (2017). *Basic Income: And How We Can Make It Happen.* Penguin.

The Migration Observatory. (2023, January). *UK Public Opinion toward Immigration: Overall Attitudes and Level of Concern.* Retrieved from https://migrationobservatory.ox.ac.uk/resources/briefings/uk-public-opinion-toward-immigration-overall-attitudes-and-level-of-concern/

Tse-Tung, M. (2018). *Quotations from Chairman Mao Tse-Tung: The Little Red Book.*